GOD CREATED ME

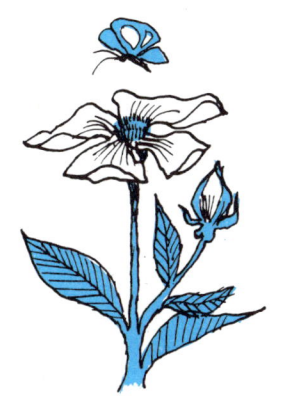

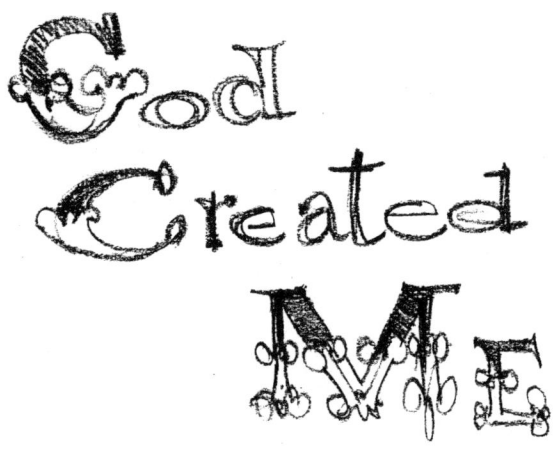

God Created Me

By Laurence Rittenhouse

Illustrated by Trina Schart Hyman

UNITED CHURCH PRESS
Boston   Philadelphia

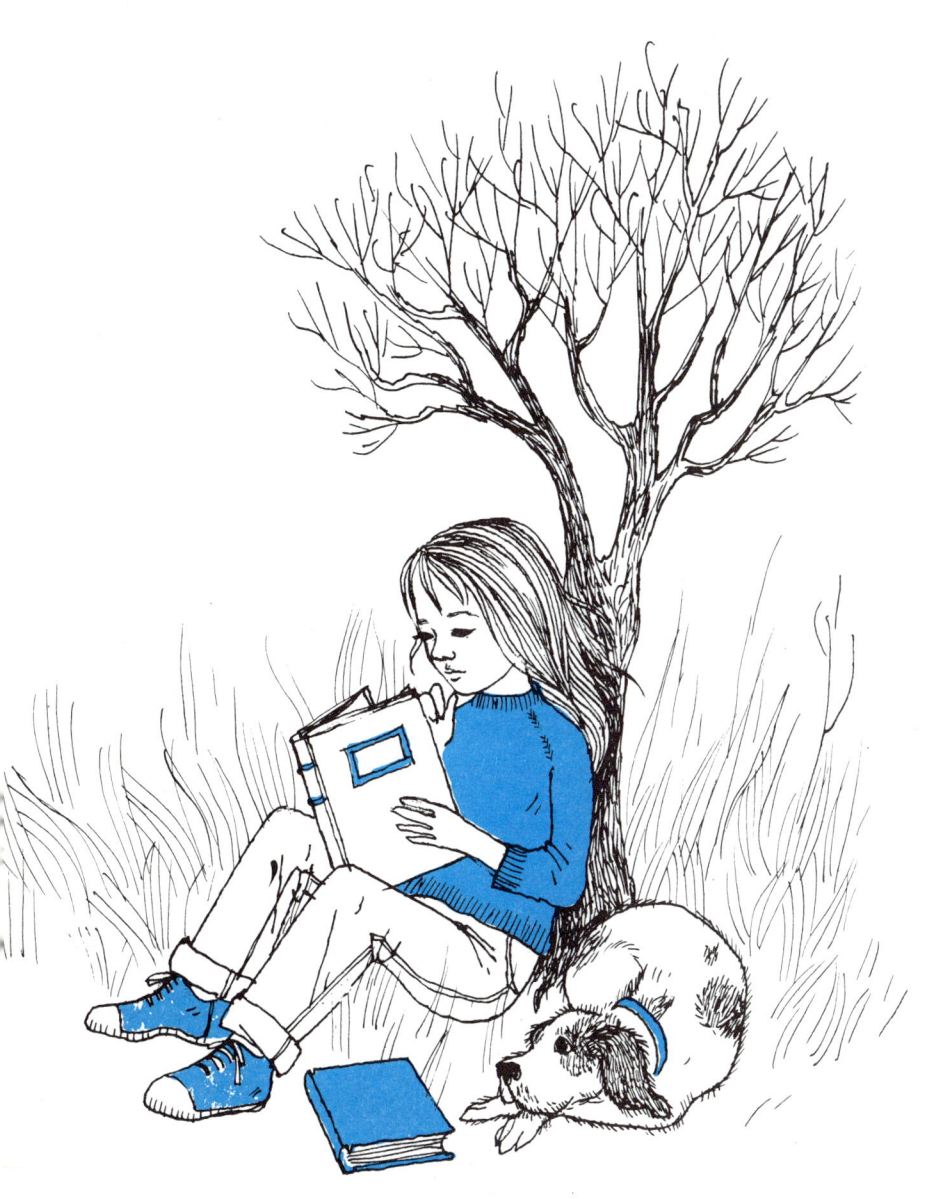

Copyright © 1963 by the United Church Press.
New Printing, 1967.

Printed in the United States of America. All rights to this book are reserved. No part of the text or illustrations may be reproduced in any form without written permission of the publishers, except brief quotations used in connection with reviews in magazines or newspapers. The scripture quotations in this publication are from the *Revised Standard Version of the Bible*, copyrighted 1946 and 1952 by the Division of Christian Education, National Council of Churches, and used by permission.

This book is part of the United Church Curriculum, prepared and published by the Division of Christian Education and the Division of Publication of the United Church Board for Homeland Ministries.

TABLE OF CONTENTS

The Person You Want to Be	7
"We Don't Like You!"	13
The Fight	21
Too Busy	27
My A+ Project	35
"Three Is a Crowd"	43
Don Makes a Discovery	48
The Outsider	61
Susy Looks for Answers	68
With God's Help	95

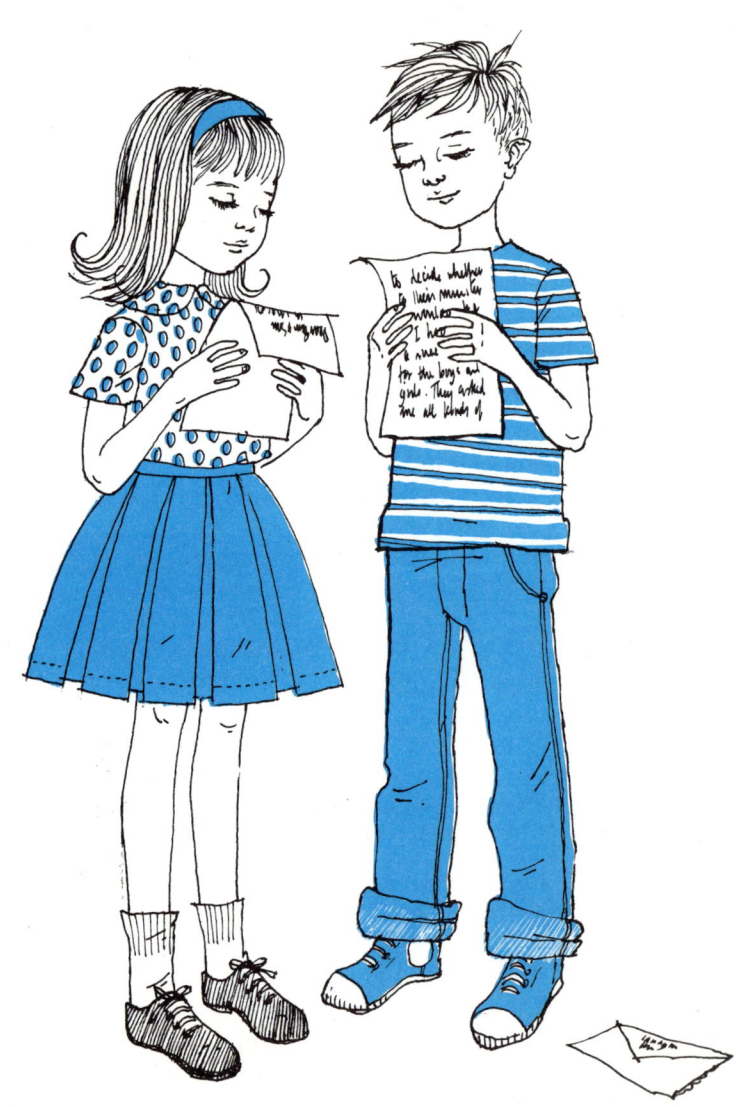

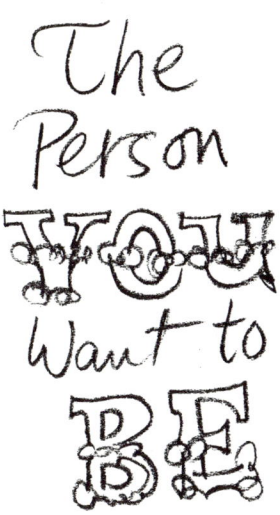

The Person You Want to Be

Dear Pam and Sam:

Hi! My name is Larry. That is not my real name, but it is what I like to be called. I like it better than my real name which is Laurence.

I am a minister, though sometimes boys and girls your age do not quite believe it. I was stopped one day in the hall of our church school by three or four boys and girls about your age. One of them said, "We thought you were a minister."

I was so surprised I did not know what to say but I finally said, "Well . . . I am!"

"But," said one of the boys, "you don't preach sermons, you don't marry people, and my dad says you never bury people."

The boys and girls were right. I do not preach sermons or marry people or conduct funerals, at least not very often. You see, I am a special kind of minister. I am a minister for boys and girls.

Once some people in a church were looking for a new minister for the boys and girls in their church. They wrote me a letter and asked me if I would visit their church to see if I might like to be the minister to their boys and girls. I did visit them and I discovered I liked the church very much.

One of the things I liked about this church was that the boys and girls helped to decide who their minister would be. I had a meeting with the boys and girls. They asked me all kinds of questions. One girl asked, "Why do you want to be a minister to boys and girls?"

My answer was this: "You and I have been created by God. It is really something when you think about

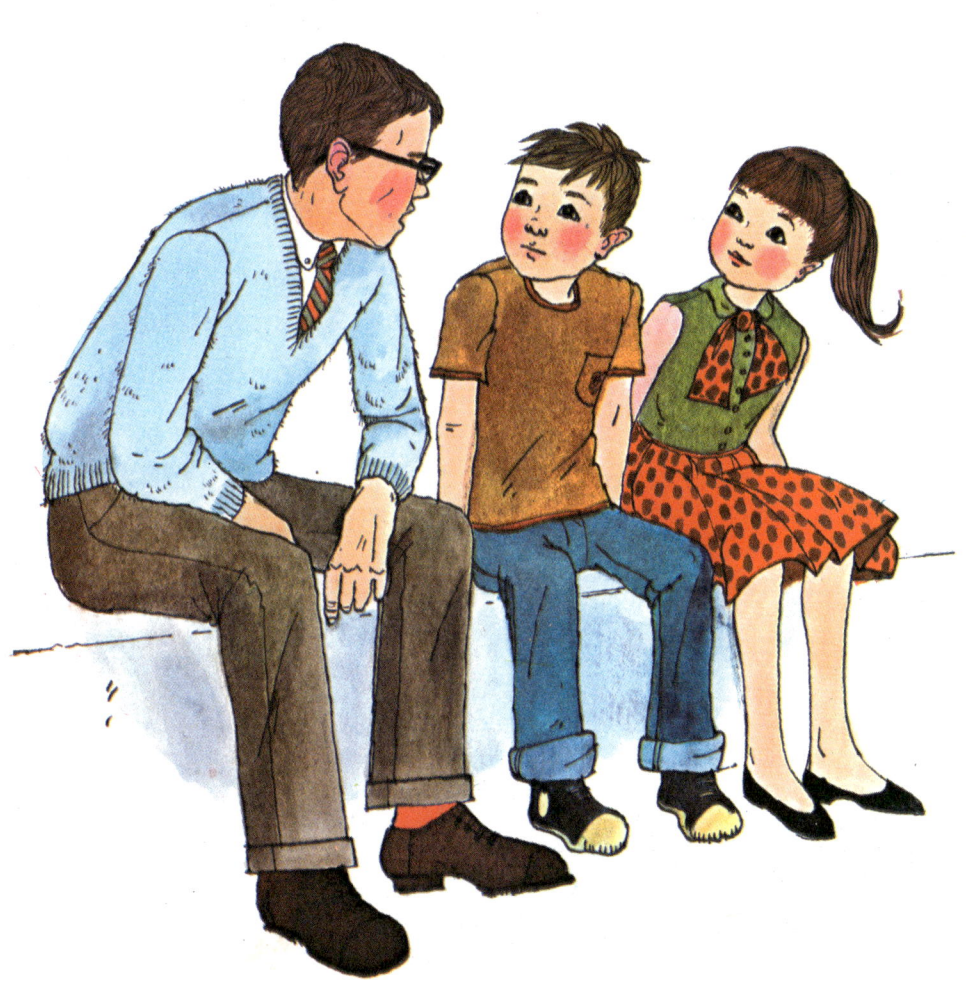

it. Imagine someone who is able to create a human being—a person—with a body that can swim, play ball, skate; a mind that can think and plan and remember; a heart (some people call it a nervous system) that can feel and love and be friendly and kind!

"What's more, God cares very, very much about us. God has not created us and then forgotten us. Instead he loves us and wants us to be the very finest persons we can become. Best of all, God helps us every day of our lives to become the finest we can become.

"But it is not only God who wants us to become the finest persons we can. Deep down inside ourselves you and I want this too. You see, there's something else about the wonderful way God created us. He made us free—free to become whatever we really want to be. So it is up to us, with God's help, to decide what kind of persons we want to be and to work hard to become that kind of person.

"This has something to do with why I want to be a minister to boys and girls. I want to help boys and girls discover the kind of persons God wants them to become.

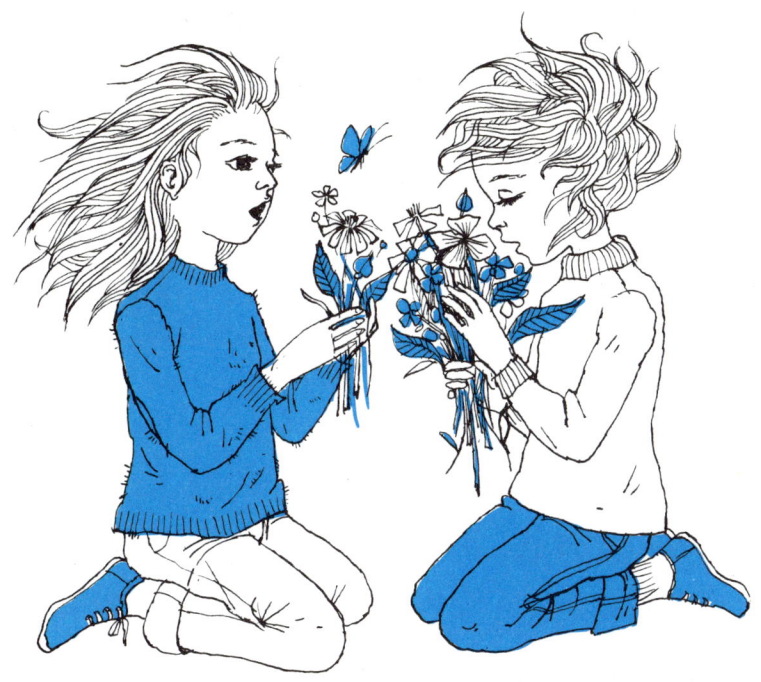

I want to help boys and girls discover the kind of persons which, deep down inside themselves, they want to be."

What kind of person do you think God wants you to be?

What kind of person do you, deep down inside, want to become?

These letters are about your answers to these two big questions. I want to tell you about the kind of person I think God wants you to become. I want to describe to you the kind of person I think you really want to be. I hope that reading these letters and stories will help you discover the kind of person God and you want you to become.

Larry

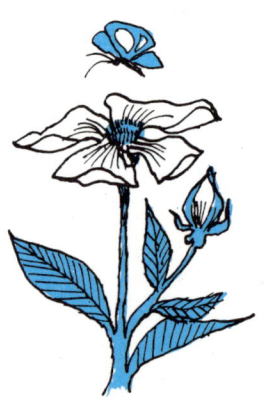

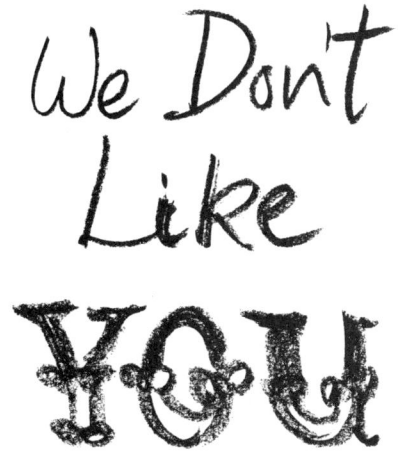

We Don't Like YOU

Dear Pam and Sam:

I think God wants you to become a person of justice.

I think you want to become a person who is fair to others.

What do I mean? Let me tell you a story about a girl named Joan. She is a friend of mine, and what happens to Joan in the story really did happen.

Joan pushed hard against the big storm door. Gradually it opened as she shoved it with all her might. Snow had tumbled down from the sky all through the night. It was piled high against the door making it hard to open.

As Joan stepped through the door she saw before her a dazzling world of white. She walked down the steps leaving deep footsteps trailing behind her. She kicked clouds of snow before her as she crossed the yard to the garage. Inside the garage, leaning against a wall, was the thing she wanted. All summer long it had stood there, ignored and useless. Now it was to become a thing of delight and fun. It was her sled.

Grabbing the rope, she pulled the sled across the cement floor of the garage. The runners screeched as they rubbed against the hard cement, but the screeching became a deep silence as Joan pulled the sled out into the snow. The runners glided quietly over the soft white blanket.

As she came to the bottom of the long hill several blocks from home, Joan looked eagerly toward the top. Joan's neighborhood friends, including Linda, whom Joan liked best of all, were already there. With great excitement Joan climbed eagerly toward the top pulling the sled behind her. Halfway up she called out, "Hi, kids!"

Reaching the top of the hill Joan could not wait another second. With a happy, "Isn't this great!" toward Linda, she plopped down her sled, fell upon it, and began the long glide toward the bottom.

Suddenly someone was beside her. She looked to her left to find Linda and her sled hardly a foot away. Without any warning Linda turned her sled toward Joan's, forcing Joan to turn quickly or be hit. "Scrunch!" Joan's sled came to a quick stop in a bank of snow at the side of the hill and Joan went rolling into the snow.

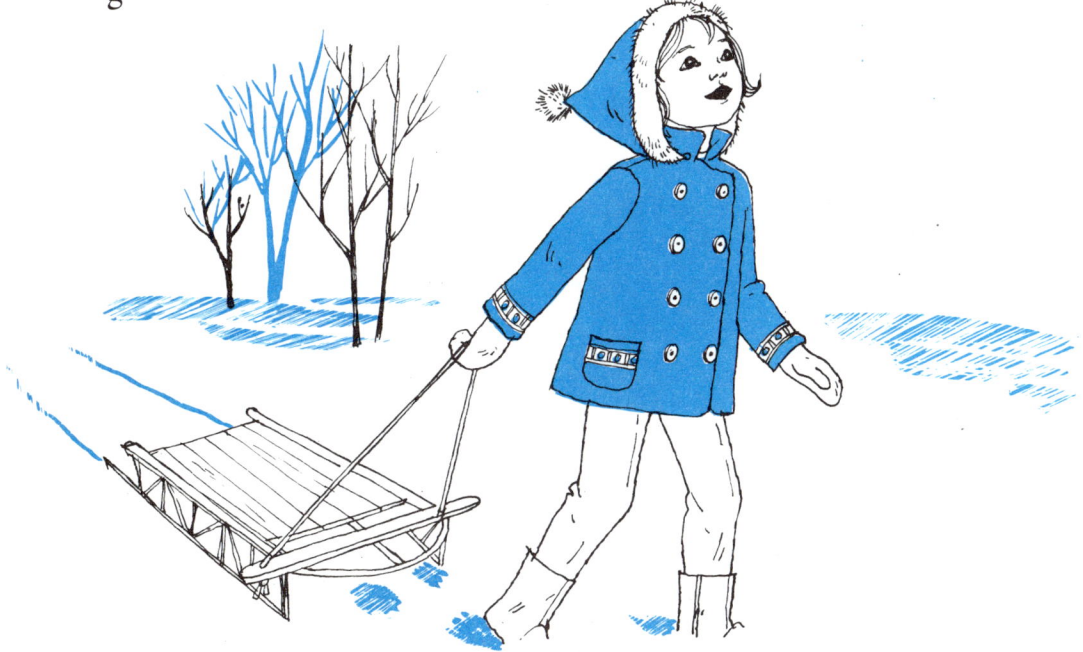

Picking herself up Joan grinned in the direction of Linda who had stopped her sled a little farther down the hill. Joan trudged the short distance back to the top. Again she plopped down her sled, fell upon it and began the exciting slide toward the bottom. Suddenly Linda was beside her again. Once more Linda turned her sled toward Joan's, forcing her to the side of the hill into the unpacked snow.

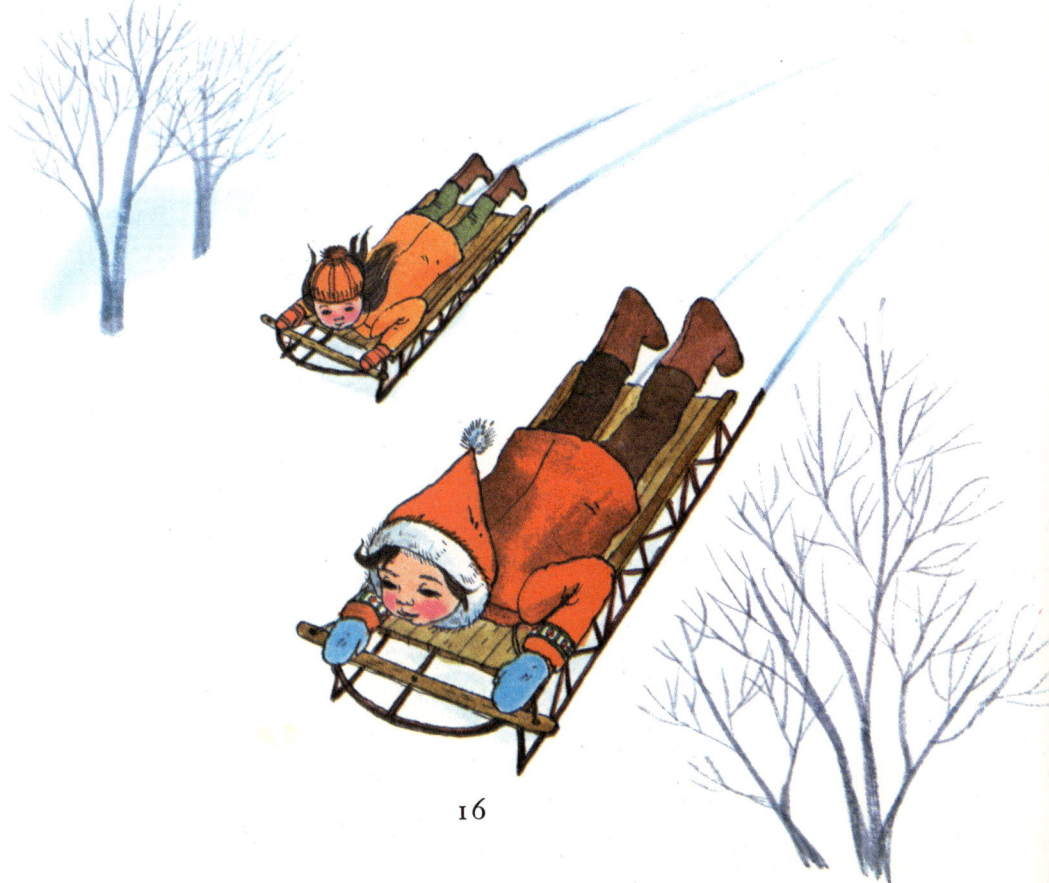

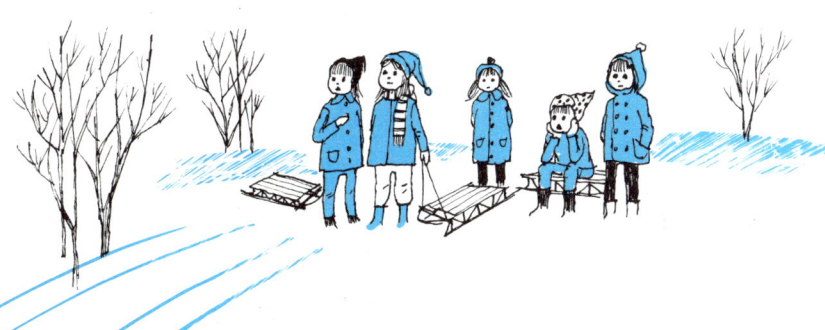

It was a little harder to grin toward Linda a second time, but Joan good-naturedly trudged up the hill and waited for Linda. As Linda reached the top Joan moved toward her to speak. Before she could say anything, ugly words leaped out at her. "Don't you get it?" shouted Linda. "We don't like you. We don't want you around today!"

The sparkle disappeared from the snow. The golden rays from the sun seemed to fade. The bright red house at the side of the hill lost its glow. Anxiously Joan's eyes darted back and forth, first toward Linda and then toward the other girls standing nearby. Waiting to hear other words, Joan tried to say something, but the sharp, ugly words leaped at her again. "We don't like you! Why don't you go home?" Linda said.

Turning away from Linda, Joan looked again toward the other girls. They did not speak but only tried to look away. The breath went out of Joan with a heavy sigh. Her shoulders drooped. Without a word she picked up her sled, carried it to the edge of the hill, laid it down gently, fell upon it, and coasted down the slope. At the bottom she reached down for the rope with which to pull the sled and walked toward home.

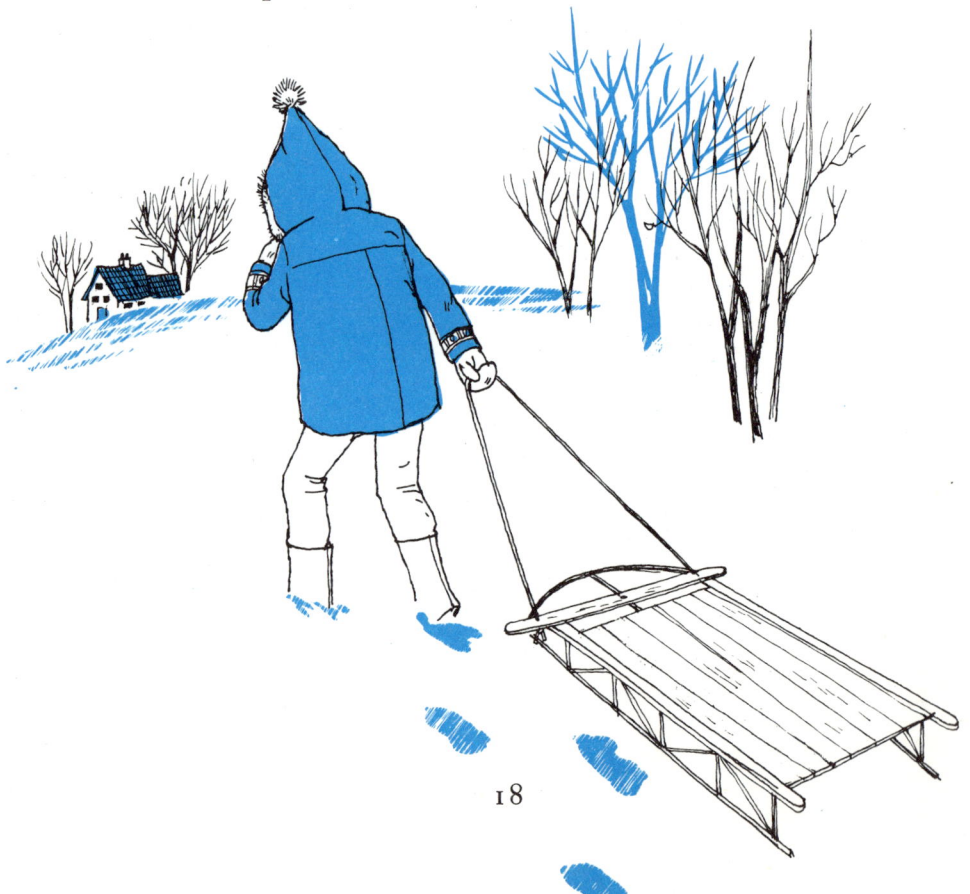

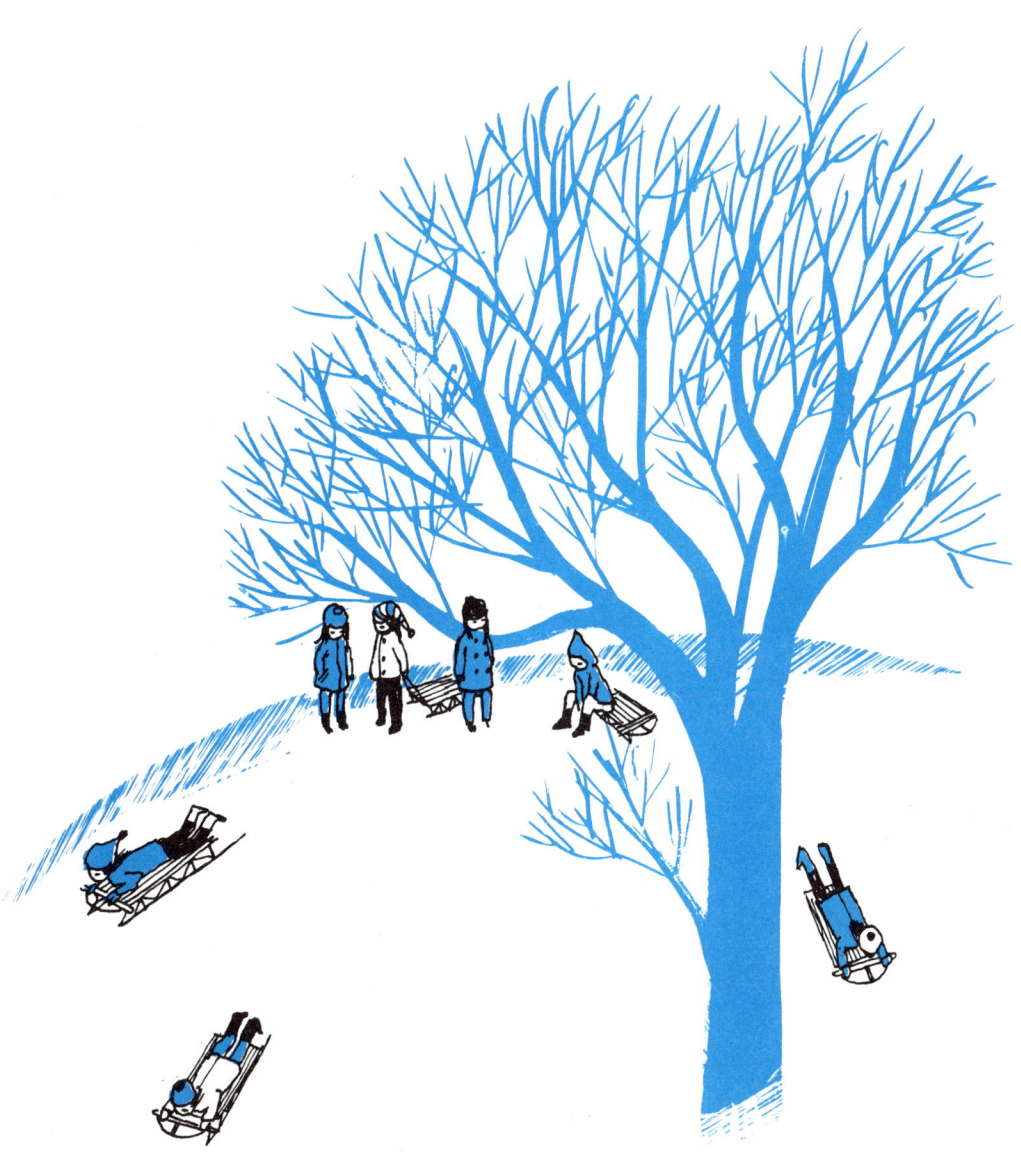

Now let's think a few minutes about being a person of justice:

A person of justice tries to feel and think how another person feels if he is treated a certain way. He tries to put himself in the other person's shoes. He does not treat the other person unjustly, or in any way that would hurt him.

Linda was not a person of justice. She treated Joan in a way that hurt her.

I think God wants you to become a fair person. I think God wants you to treat other people in a way that will not hurt them. I think that deep down inside yourself you want to be a fair person. I think you really want to treat people in a way that will not hurt them.

I hope you become a person of justice!

Larry

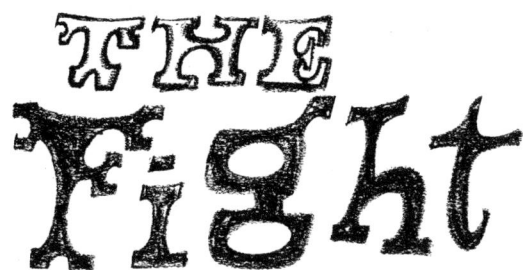

THE Fight

Dear Pam and Sam:

I think God wants you to become a person of power.

I think deep down inside yourself you want to become a person of power.

What do I mean?

When I was in the fourth grade, my best friend was a boy named Frank. I had met Frank three years before when we were in the first grade. Almost from the first day we were the best of pals. We sat next to each other in school when our teachers would let us. We walked home together after school. Sometimes on Friday nights we stayed overnight at each other's houses. We went to the movies together Saturday afternoon. We went to the same church school on Sunday morning. When Christmas came along each year we gave each other presents. Frank and I were always together.

Then one day several other boys tried to get Frank and me to fight each other. I don't know why. Maybe they thought it would be fun to see two such good friends get into a real fight. Day after day they would shout, "Larry's afraid to fight!" or "Frank's scared of Larry!" Sometimes they would make up lies about mean things Frank said about me. Sometimes they would tell Frank that I didn't like him any more.

Then one day they told me that Frank said he would fight me, but that I was afraid. That was enough for me! I told the boys they should tell Frank that I would be on a certain corner after school, and that if he wasn't too scared, I would fight him.

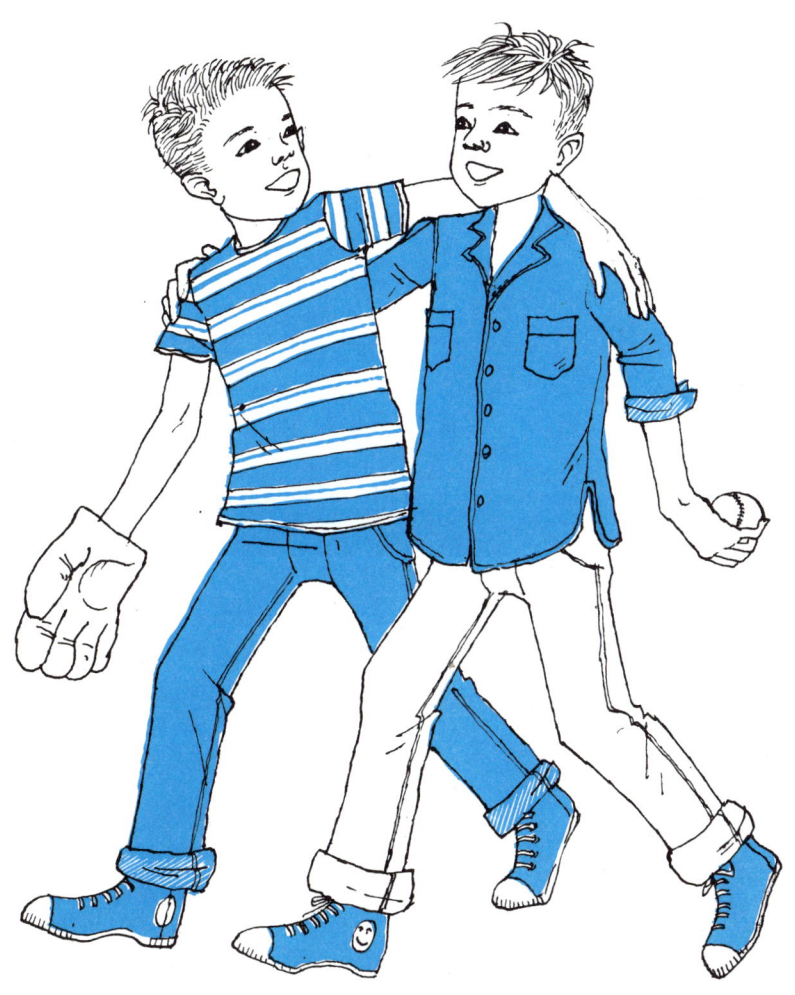

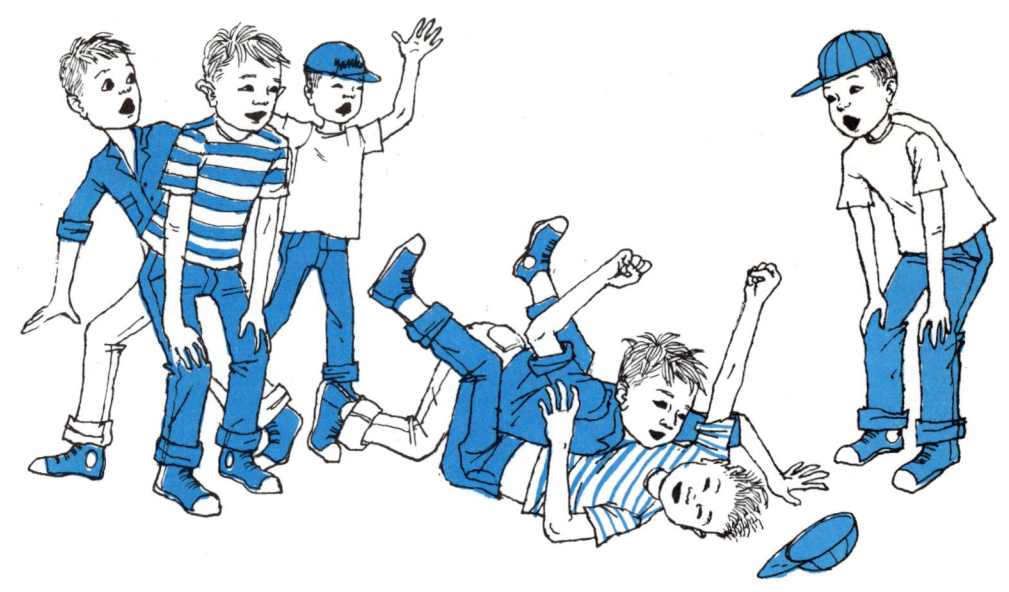

After school I waited on the corner. It was about two blocks from school so we would not get caught by the teachers or the principal. There was a big red house on the corner with a wide green lawn in front of it. Frank did not come right away. I think I was hoping he would not come at all. I wasn't scared of Frank but I did not want to fight him. After all, he was my best friend.

I was turning to go home when I saw Frank and about four other boys coming down the street. They came to the cor-

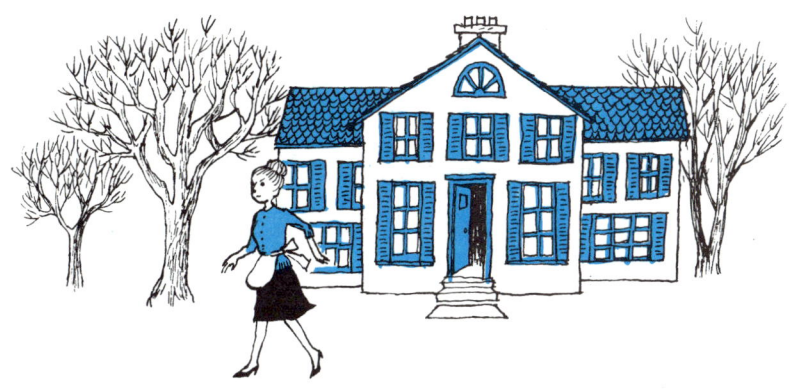

ner where I was standing. Even before Frank could put down his books one of the boys pushed him into me and shouted, "Fight!" All of the other boys shouted too. Some said, "Come on, Larry, poke him!" Others said, "Come on, Frank, hit him good!" We did too! We hit and pushed and scratched and shoved and sometimes rolled over and over on the big green lawn. We were not really hurting each other, however. I guess we were not mad enough. I think each of us wished he could quit without being called a sissy by the other boys.

Then something lucky happened. At least I thought it was lucky. The lady who owned the yard in which we were fighting came out and chased us all away. I went to my house and Frank went to his. I don't know what became of the other boys.

Now, what has all of this to do with being a person of power?

A person of power is one who decides for himself what he is going to do in a certain situation. Of course he listens to what other people think he should do. Finally, however, he decides for himself.

When I got into a fight with Frank I was not a person of power. I did not really want to fight Frank. Inside myself I felt only friendship for Frank. If I had decided for myself what I should do, I would not have fought Frank.

But I did not decide for myself. I let the other boys decide for me. I let them talk me into something I did not want to do. I was not a person of power.

I think God wants you to become a person of power. I think God wants you to decide for yourself what you are going to do in certain situations. I think that deep down inside yourself you want to become a person of power. You really want to decide for yourself what you are going to do in certain situations.

I hope you become a person of power.

Larry

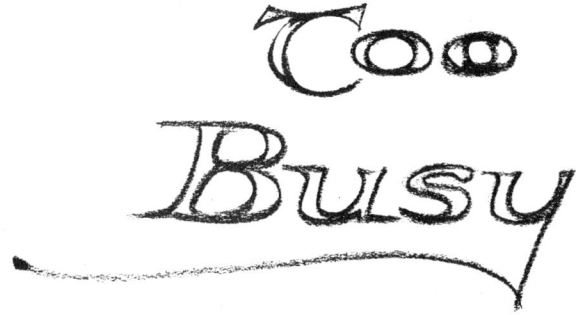

Too Busy

Dear Pam and Sam:

    I think God wants you to become a person who can put yourself in another's place.

    I think you want to become a person who can think what it would be like to be in another's place.

    Sometimes the person you need to think about is close by, as near as in your home.

"Oh, Mother, why does Margie have to come tomorrow?" Carol sounded very cross. "I'll be packing to go to Girl Scout camp, and I can't bother with her!"

"Carol, stop a minute," Mrs. Walker said, "think what you're saying! You know Uncle Dick has to go to England on business this summer and that Aunt Miriam is going with him because the doctor said the trip would help her to get her strength back after her operation. We're glad to have Margie stay with us for the summer!"

"Maybe you're glad, but I'm not!" said Carol. She stamped noisily out of the room.

Ever since last summer Carol had been planning on going to Girl Scout camp for the month of July with Betty who lived next door. Betty had gone last year, but Carol was not quite old enough to be a Scout then. She could not go to Girl Scout camp.

All year long Carol had been saving her money to help pay for camp. She had known the Girl Scout oath since last summer. For months she had been studying for her tenderfoot tests. Finally, in May, her tenth birthday came, just in time for her to take and pass the tests. For a week now she had been packing her suitcase and unpacking it each night. It was a nuisance to have to bother with Margie, who was only nine years old.

Mother talked with Carol again before she went to bed, but Carol was no happier about the whole thing. All she could think of was herself, her own plans.

When Carol came home from school the next day, Margie was there.

"Hi, Carol," said Margie, "I've been waiting ages for you."

"Hi," said Carol, in a low voice. "I'll be too busy to play with you tonight."

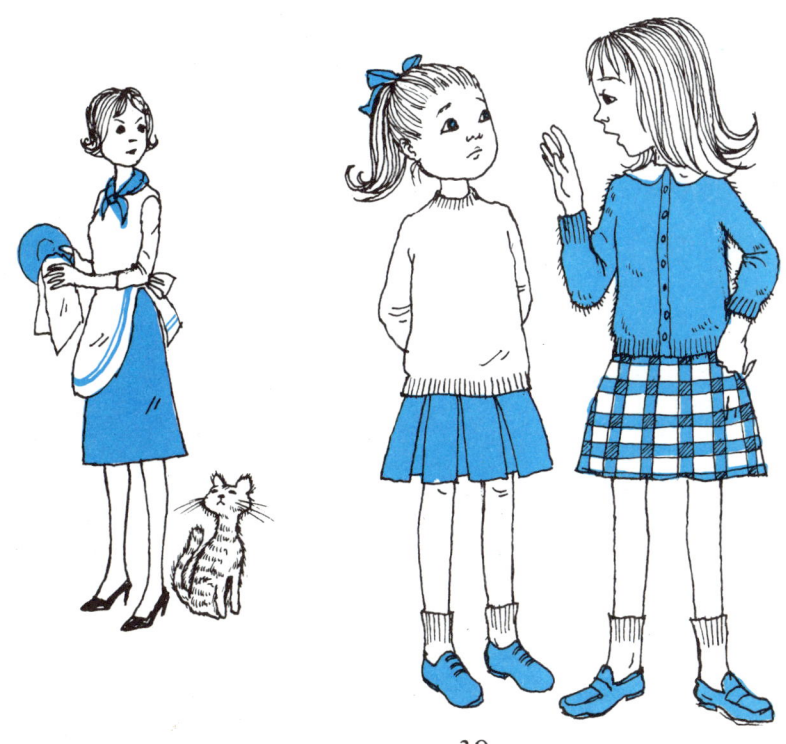

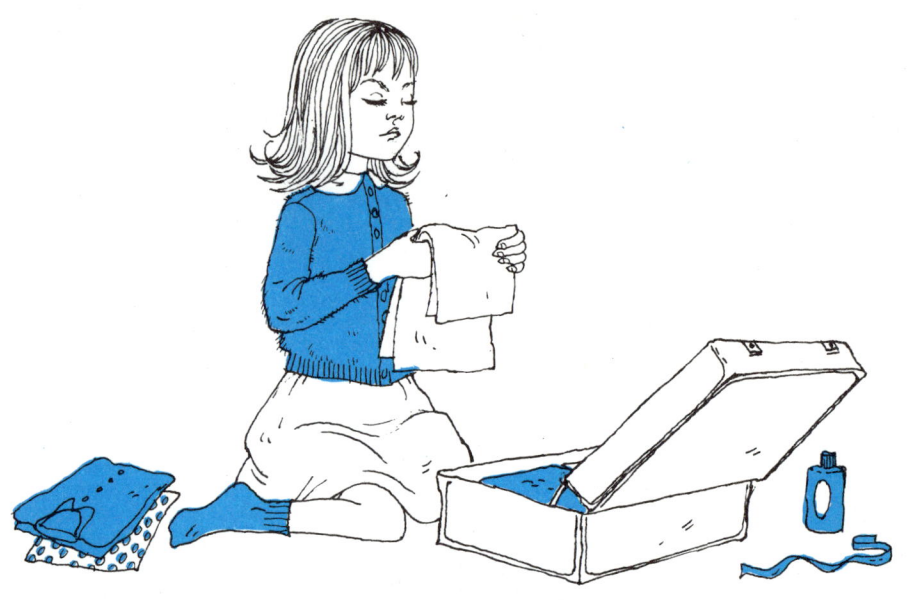

"Why?" asked Margie.

"Because Betty and I are going to Girl Scout camp on Saturday for two weeks. I have to go over to Betty's house to talk about our plans and when I come home I'll be packing."

Margie looked from Carol to her aunt. "Why can't I go to camp too? I'm a Brownie."

"Brownies can't go at the same time the Girl Scouts go. They have a different time. Besides, all the places are taken for the first camping period," said Carol scornfully.

"Never mind, Margie," said her aunt, "I'm going out now to do some errands and to pick up your uncle at the train. Come along and be company for me."

"All right," said Margie in a sad little voice.

While Carol was at camp, Margie found a friend her own age in the next block. Her name was Janet. They had a good time together, but Margie kept thinking about Carol. Why had she been so mean to her? Perhaps it was only because she was so excited about going to camp. When Carol and Betty came back they would all play together. There would be lots to hear about the girls' fun at camp. Probably they would know some good new games to play.

At last the day came when the girls were to return. The bus bringing all the campers would arrive at Girl Scout headquarters at two o'clock. Mrs. Walker was going to meet it and bring Carol and Betty home.

"Would you and Janet like to meet the bus with me this afternoon?" she asked Margie.

"I would," said Margie, "and I know Janet would too. I'll call her right now and find out if she can go."

Janet's answer was "Yes," and the girls went off with Mrs. Walker to meet the Girl Scout bus.

It was exciting to see the bus come in. The girls were very gay. They were singing some of the songs they had learned while they were at camp.

Carol ran to her mother, hugged her tightly, and said, "Oh, Mother, I'm so glad to see you! Camp was so much fun. May I go next year? May I?" She didn't even seem to see Margie.

In a few minutes the luggage was sorted out and Carol and Betty had found their suitcases and bedrolls. They climbed into the back seat of the car. Margie and Janet got in front.

"Carol, I haven't heard you say a word to Margie. Margie dear, introduce your new friend to Carol and Betty," said Mrs. Walker.

"Oh, hello, Margie," said Carol.

Margie introduced Janet to the bigger girls, and waited for them to tell all about the exciting times they had had at camp. But Carol and Betty were very busy talking to each other. Their voices were low, and what they were saying could not be heard by those on the front seat. Every few sentences they would burst out laughing.

And that's the way it went when they were back home. The two big girls always had some important plan to carry out. Margie and Janet just weren't included.

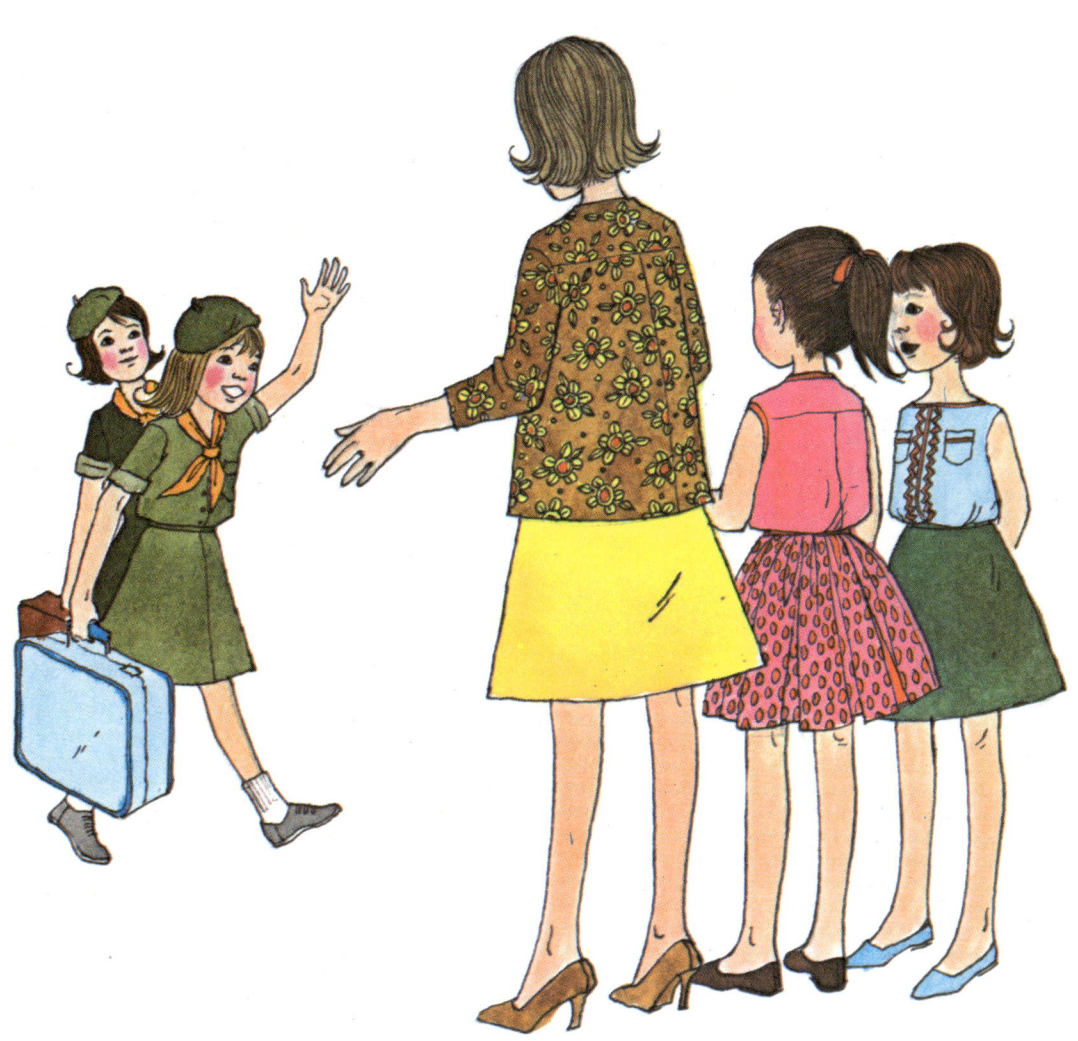

Carol had not learned to put herself in another's place. She did not think what it would be like to be Margie, and be left out of everything. She didn't remember what it felt like to have the older girls forget you were around.

I think God wants you to be a person who can put himself in another's place. I think you want to be a person who can think what it would be like to be in another's place.

Larry

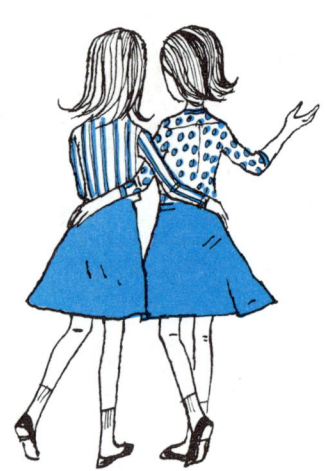

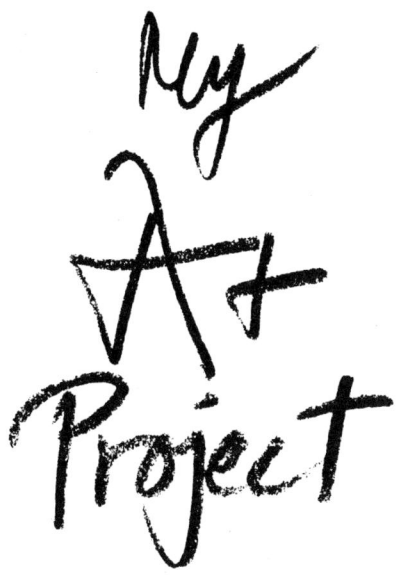

Dear Pam and Sam:

    I think God wants you to become a creative person.

    I think that deep down inside yourself you want to become a creative person.

    What do I mean?

When I was in the fourth grade we began to study things about other countries. We learned a little bit about what happened in these countries long ago. We learned something about how people live in these countries today.

Near the end of the year each boy and girl was to make a special project about one of the countries we had studied. It could be a scrapbook or a poster. It might be a table scene showing

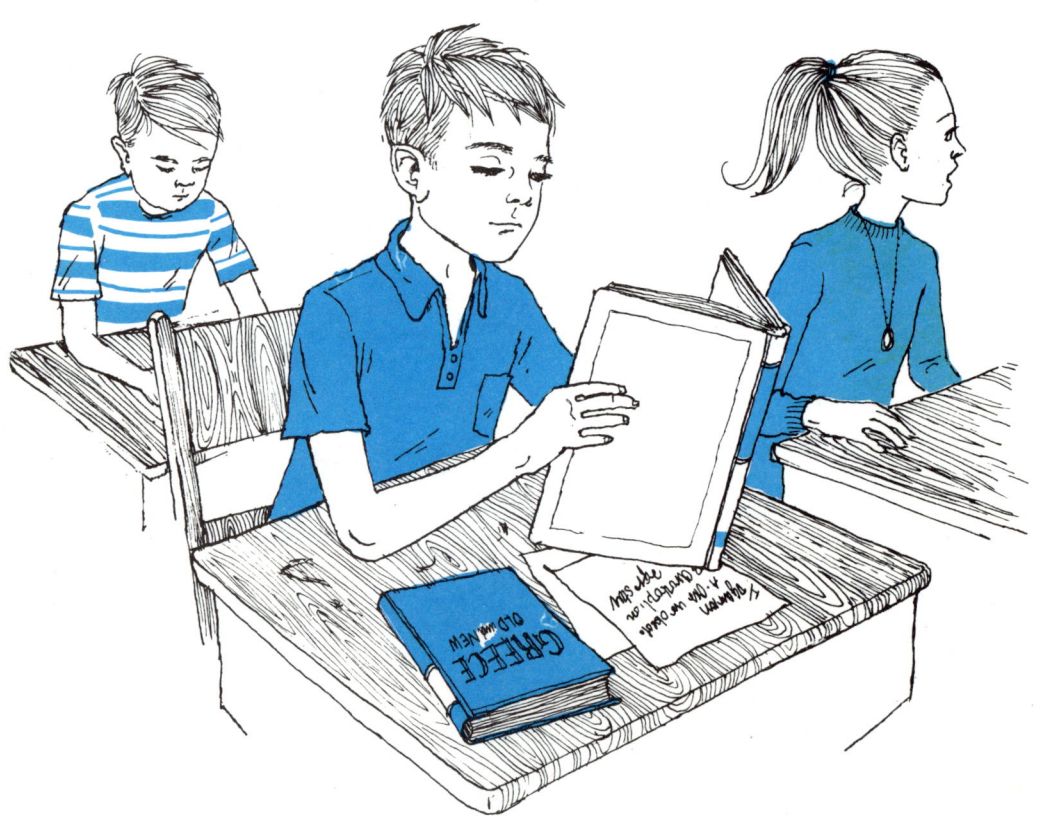

something in that country. It might even be a story.

I decided I wanted to make something very different and unusual. I thought and thought about what country I should choose and what I should make. For some reason I chose Greece. But what should the project be? I looked through books about Greece. I looked up information about Greece in the *World Book*. I talked with my teacher about Greece. I even went to see a man in my town who had lived in Greece.

All of a sudden I had an idea. It came to me one afternoon when I was in school. I was looking at a book about Greece when I saw a picture of three kinds of Greek columns.

You know what columns are. They are the tall round posts in front of some large buildings. If you have ever seen pictures of our nation's Capitol in Washington you know that there are columns in front of it. Many churches have columns in front of them also.

Anyway, a long time ago in Greece there were three kinds of columns. They were called Doric, Ionic, and Corinthian. Each kind of column had a different kind of decoration, or what was called a *capital*, at the top. The Doric was a very simple top, the Ionic less simple, and the Corinthian capital was quite fancy.

As I was looking at the picture a question popped into my

head. Were there Doric, Ionic, and Corinthian columns in my home town? I could hardly wait until school was out for the day. I dashed home, told Mom what I wanted to find out and ran toward downtown.

I lived in Washington, D.C., so the first place I went was to the capitol building. I looked up at the huge columns in front of the Capitol and jumped with excitement. They were Corinthian columns. Quickly I ran across the park, down a street, and was soon looking up at the Supreme Court building. Hurrah! Ionic columns! All I needed now were Doric columns and my idea for a project would work.

I ran to the post office. More Ionic columns. I went to a church. No columns at all. I went to an office building. No columns there either. Then I remembered. There was a big funeral home not far from my house. There were columns there, of that I was sure. I dashed down three streets to the funeral home. It was a huge building that used to be someone's private home. Anxiously I looked up at the big white columns. DORIC!

Imagine! All three kinds of Greek columns on buildings right in my own home town. Greece was a long distance from my home but the ideas for the capitals on these buildings had come from across the ocean. Now I was ready to go ahead with my project.

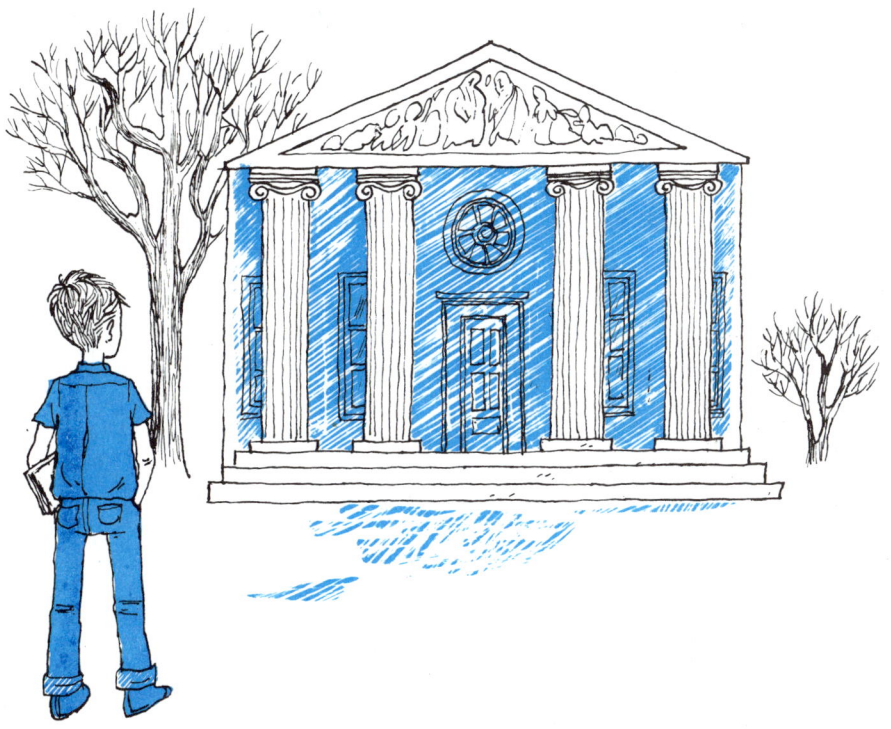

The next Saturday was a bright sunshiny day. I borrowed my folks' camera, asked my dad for some money, and headed for the drugstore. There I bought a roll of film.

After the man at the drugstore helped me to put the film in the camera I walked as quickly as I could to the Capitol. Click! Click! I had two pictures of Corinthian columns. Then I went to the Supreme Court building to get pictures of the Ionic columns. Back through the business district and a few blocks farther east brought me to the funeral home. Click! Click! Two pictures of Doric columns.

On the way home I took two pictures of just anything in order to use up the roll of film. At first I planned to take the film to a drugstore and have it developed. Then the thought came to me, "Why not develop it myself?" I took it home and laid it away for a week or two until I could learn how to make prints from the film.

Then I started to read about how to develop film. I read about darkrooms and sinks, water taps and trays, basins and jars of chemicals. I read about *developers* and *stop baths* and *hypos*. I read about *negatives* and *positives*.

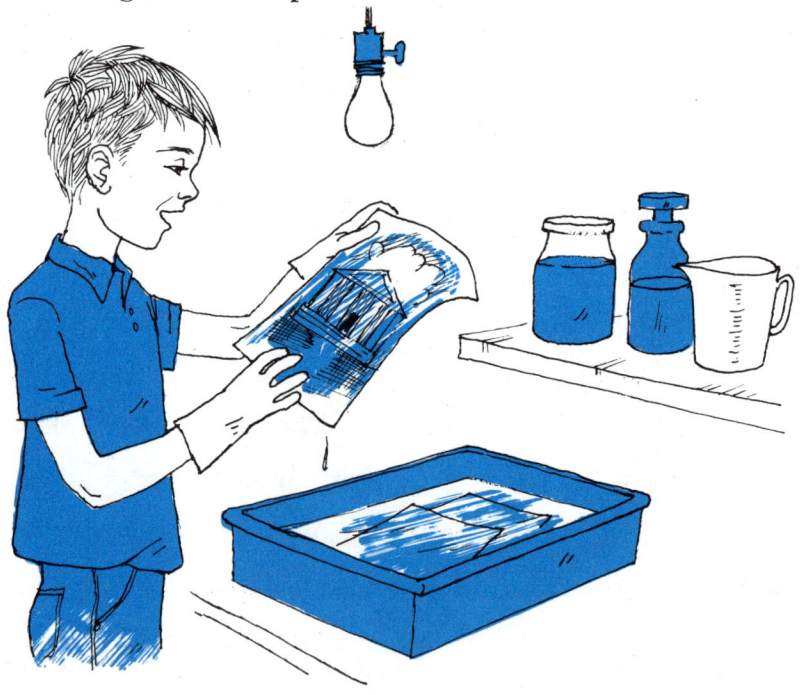

In a few weeks I had set up a darkroom in an old coalbin in our basement. I took pictures of friends and of our house and other places around town. I developed these in order to learn how. Then one day I made prints from my film with the pictures of the columns. They came out just right!

The next evening I mounted the three best pictures—one of each kind of column—on a big sheet of gray poster paper. At the top in large black letters I wrote the words GREEK COLUMNS IN OUR CITY. On the back of the poster I pasted two sheets of paper. On the paper was a story of how I took the pictures and developed them myself. The next day I took the poster to school and gave it to my teacher.

One day a week or so later our teacher suddenly said, "Oh yes, I want to give your projects on other countries back to you today." I could hardly wait as she called off our names and each of us went up to her table to get his project. Finally it was my turn. She said nothing as she handed it to me, but I found she had written on the back, "A most creative project! A+!"

I had been a creative person.

A creative person is one who feels and thinks until from inside himself he makes something new. He does not copy what someone else has already done. He makes something new from which he and other people can learn. He makes something new for people to enjoy or to use. This is what I did when I made my poster about Greek columns.

God did not make each of us to be creative in exactly the same way. Some boys and girls are creative with their hands: they are creative in their work with paints or wood or clay. Some are creative with their minds: they write stories or compose music, or they make scientific discoveries. Some are creative in the way they live with others: they are happy and thoughtful. They make others glad.

I think God wants you to become a creative person. I think God wants you to feel and think until from inside yourself you make something new.

I think you want to be a creative person. I think that deep down inside yourself you want to feel and think until you yourself make something new.

I hope you become a creative person!

Larry

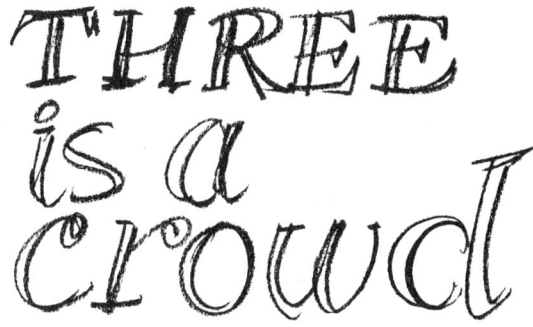
Three is a crowd

Dear Pam and Sam:

I think God wants you to become a person who trusts other people.

I think that deep down inside yourself you want to become a person who trusts other people.

What do I mean?

I know a girl who never trusts another person. She thinks other people are trying to run her life. She thinks other people are always trying to get the best of her, trying to use her to get what they want for themselves. She never really believes another person is trying to do something good for her.

This girl has good reasons for feeling this way. Let me tell you about the kind of thing that keeps happening to her. Her name is Barbara.

It was Wednesday afternoon and Barbara was furious. Her best friend Leslie, who had moved away from Chicago six months ago, was visiting Barbara for two days during spring vacation. Leslie had arrived in Chicago that morning and the two girls were planning to go to the movies together that afternoon. They were having fun getting acquainted again and talking over old times. Leslie wanted to hear about all her old friends and what they were doing. Barbara wanted to hear about the things Leslie did in her new home town. It was wonderful for best friends to be together again.

Around noon Mary called to ask Barbara to go to the movies with her that afternoon. Barbara explained that she and Leslie were going. Barbara would go with Mary some other time.

Everything was fine until an hour later when Mary's mother called up Barbara's mother and said, "Barbara certainly was not very nice to Mary. She wouldn't let Mary go to the movies with Leslie and her."

Barbara's mother replied, "I'm certain Barbara did not mean it that way. You tell Mary I'll stop by and pick her up about two o'clock when I drive Barbara and Leslie to the movie. It will be much more fun for all three of them to go together."

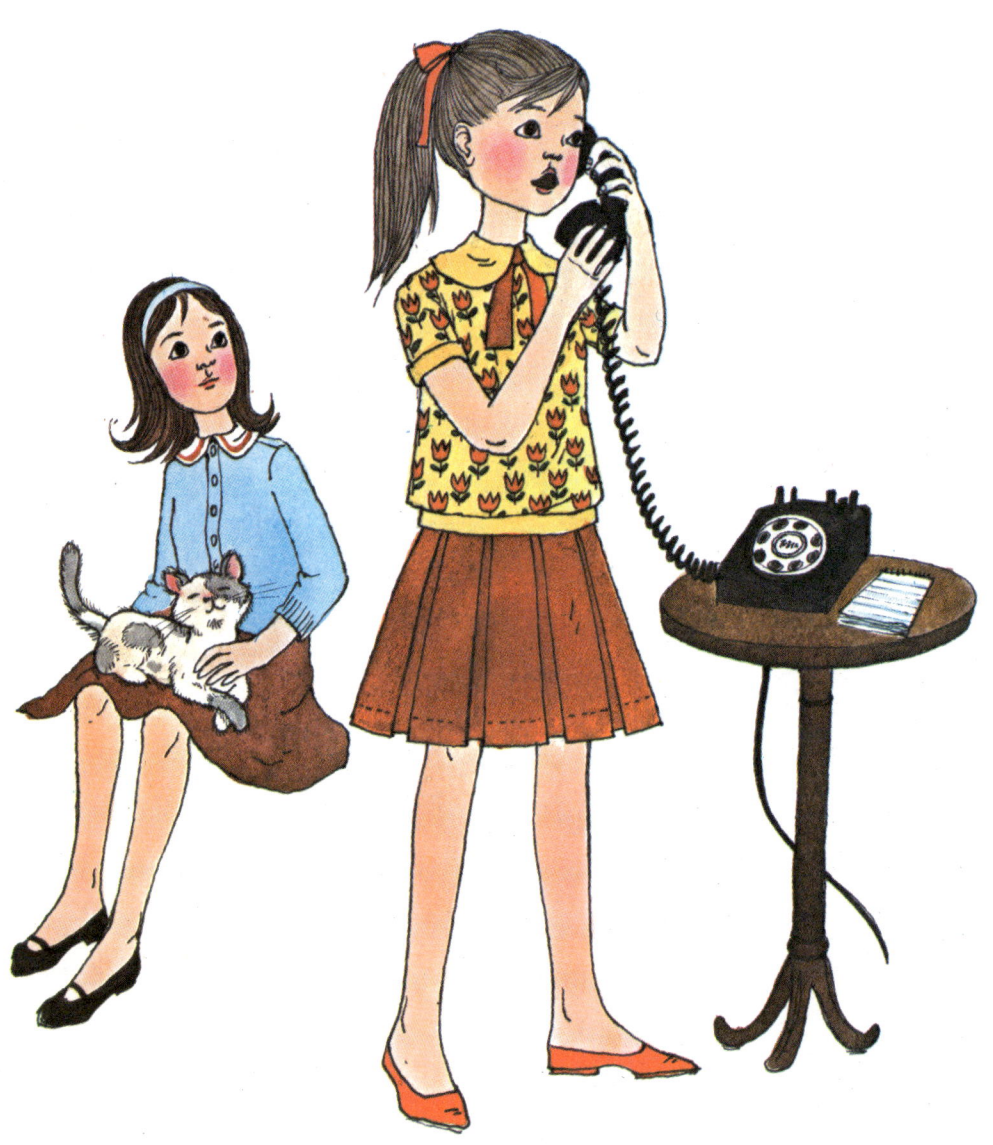

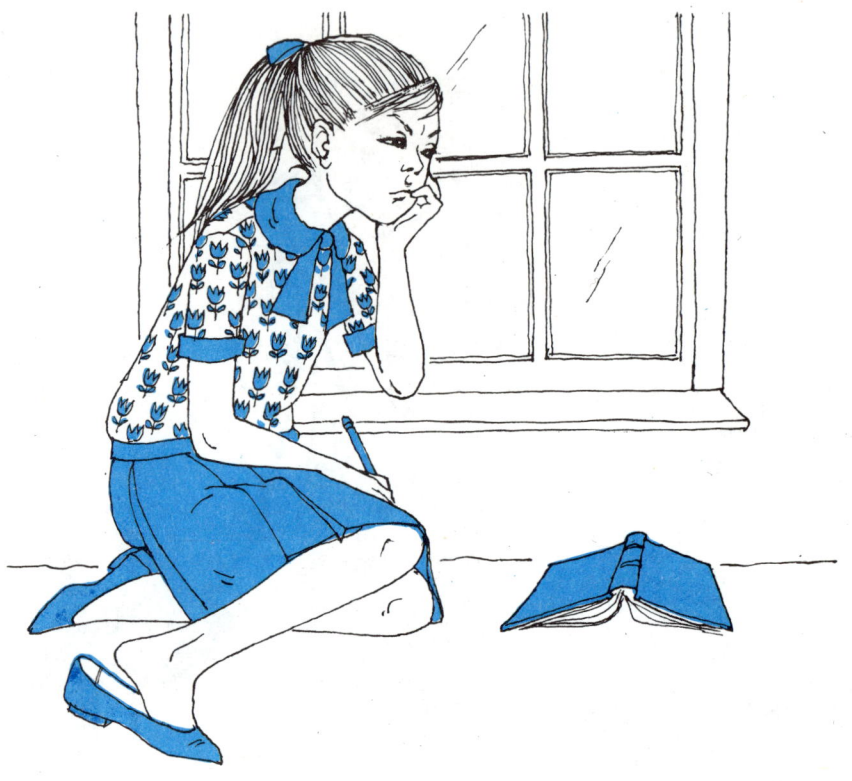

When Barbara told me several days later what had happened to her, she was just as furious as she was when it happened Wednesday afternoon. "This is always happening to me," said Barbara. "My mom always interferes and decides things for me. People are always trying to run my life. They don't think about how I feel. They only think about what they think I should do. I don't trust anybody."

Barbara had good reasons for feeling this way. Her mother did interfere again and again. Barbara could never decide anything for herself without being afraid it might be changed.

I hope that most of the people you know are people who can be trusted. I hope they are people who care about you, who try to understand how you feel when you are treated in a certain way.

I think God wants you to become a person who trusts other people.

I think you want to be a person who trusts other people.

I hope you are becoming a person who trusts other people.

Larry

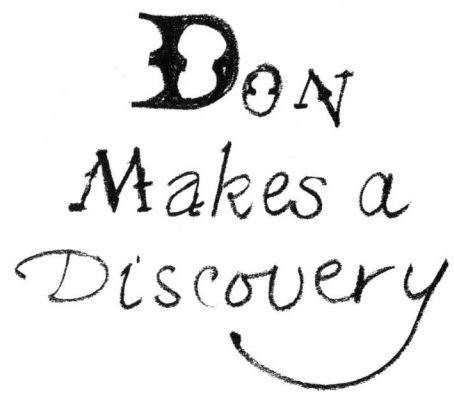
Don Makes a Discovery

Dear Pam and Sam:

    I think God wants us to use our minds to do all the wonderful things a person can learn to do.

    I think that you want to use your own mind to do all the wonderful things you can learn to do.

    I knew a boy once who thought he wanted to find an easy way to do this. Let me tell you about Don.

"Possible," said Miss Crandall. "If you work hard, it is *possible* to do many things."

"World," said Miss Crandall. "Columbus discovered the *world* was round."

"Believe," said Miss Crandall. "I *believe* today is Tuesday."

The spelling lesson droned on in the fourth-grade classroom of Westfield School. Twenty-seven pairs of eyes looked up toward the voice that pronounced each word and used it in a sentence. Twenty-seven pairs of eyes looked down at twenty-seven sheets of white paper—one sheet in front of each pair. Carefully twenty-seven hands made the letters that, put together in a continuous line, spelled a word.

For once Don was glad his last name was Williams. Since it began with a "W," he almost always had a seat near the back of the room. Last year in the third grade his teacher had decided the "W's" and the "Y's" and the "Z's" should have the seats up front. But that was last year. This year Don was in his more usual position near the back of the room.

"Possible," thought Don. "Does that end with 'bel' or 'ble'?" Cautiously he looked down on the seat of his chair. He moved his leg ever so slightly—just enough for him to be able to see the top half of page forty-two in his spelling book. There it

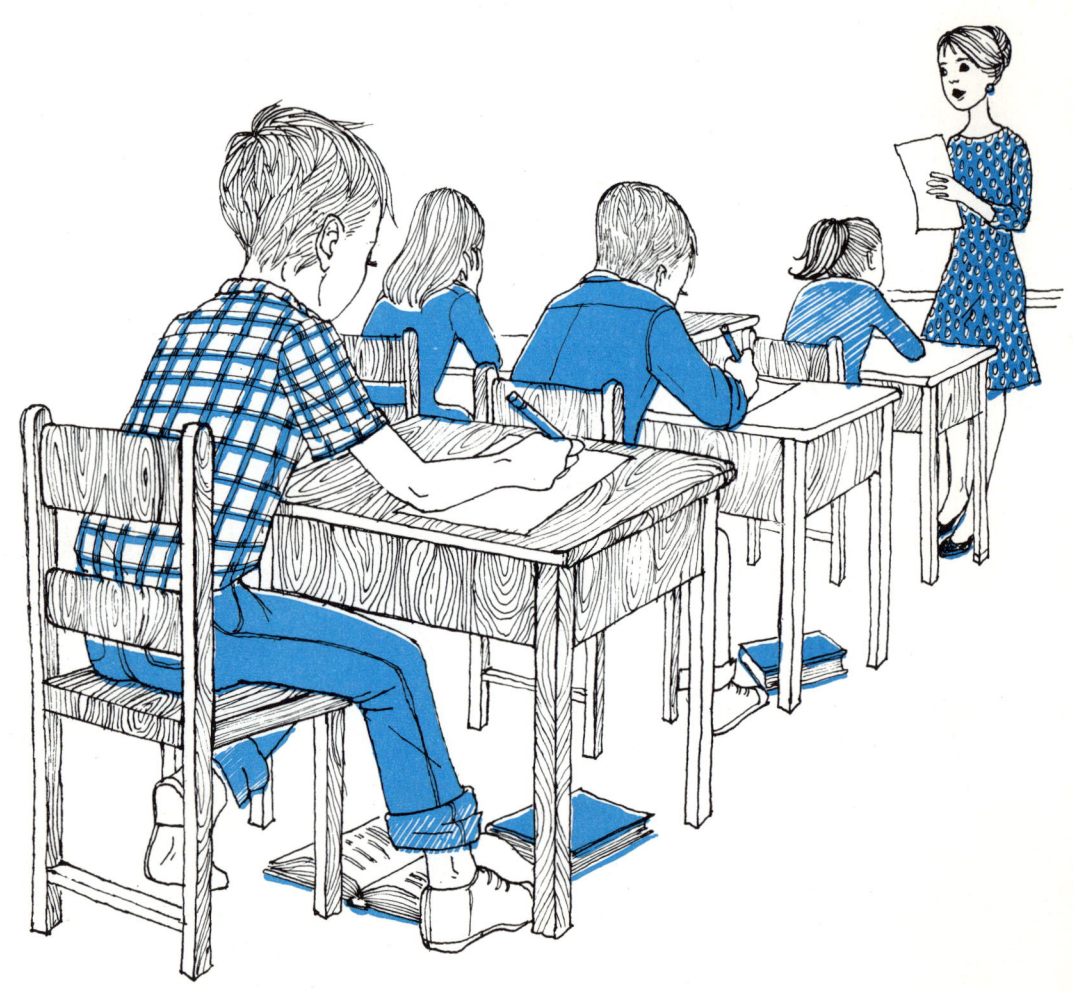

was—the fourth word down in the second column: "possible—p-o-s-s-i-b-l-e."

"World," thought Don. "That's easy. Just like in World Series."

"Believe," thought Don. " 'I' before 'E' except after—or is it 'E' before 'I'?" Cautiously he looked down again at the book under his leg.

Don was glad Miss Crandall decided to read a story to the class during the last twenty minutes of the afternoon. It would have been hard after the spelling test to concentrate on anything else. "Well, why is it so wrong to cheat?" mumbled Don. "How does anybody really know what is right and wrong?"

On that particular afternoon Don did not wait for any of the friends with whom he usually walked. He did not stop to watch the giant gasoline truck fill the underground tanks at the corner gas station. He did not stop to see the rattling sheets of tin being unloaded at the tin shop directly behind the grocery store. Instead, walking home slowly while hardly looking to the right or the left, he almost went past the white stone steps in front of his home.

"What shall I do?" thought Don.

He had felt bad almost as soon as the spelling test was over, but he probably would have been able to push his feelings away if it had not been for Marjorie. As he reached for his coat in his locker next to Marjorie's, she had turned to him and said, "I saw you look at your spelling book. I'm going to tell."

"Tattletale!" he had retorted.

"I don't care, I'm going to," she had replied.

"Girls!" thought Don as he trudged on home. "Always telling the teacher."

A thousand thoughts went through Don's mind as he walked. What should he do? If Marjorie told Miss Crandall, she would probably tell his parents. He was afraid of what would happen, though he did not have any idea what his parents would do. He had never before been in this kind of trouble. Maybe Miss Crandall would not tell, but she would probably give him a low grade. Then his parents would know something had happened.

"Anyway," thought Don, "I don't want a low grade."

If only he had not cheated. But what else could be done? He had forgotten all about the spelling test. When he remembered it at the last minute, he'd had to do something. His folks always

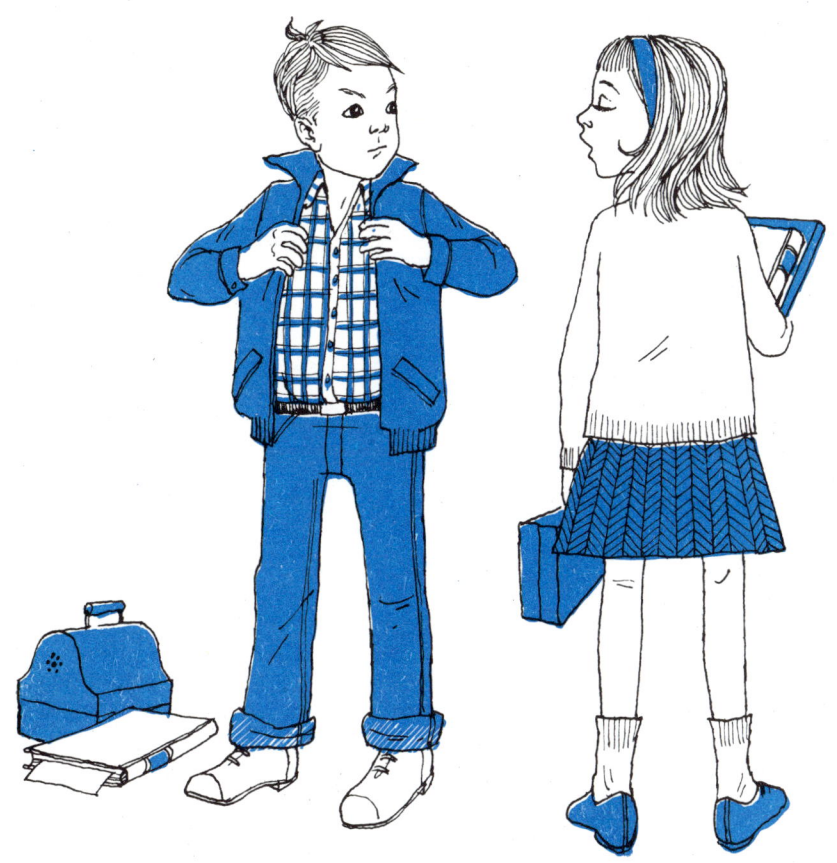

wanted him to make good grades. If he did not make an "A" on the spelling test, he did not know what they would say.

"Why is it wrong to cheat?" Don asked himself. "How do you decide what is right and what is wrong? Dad and Mom say it's wrong to cheat. Mom is always getting after the butcher at the grocery store because he gives an ounce or two less meat than

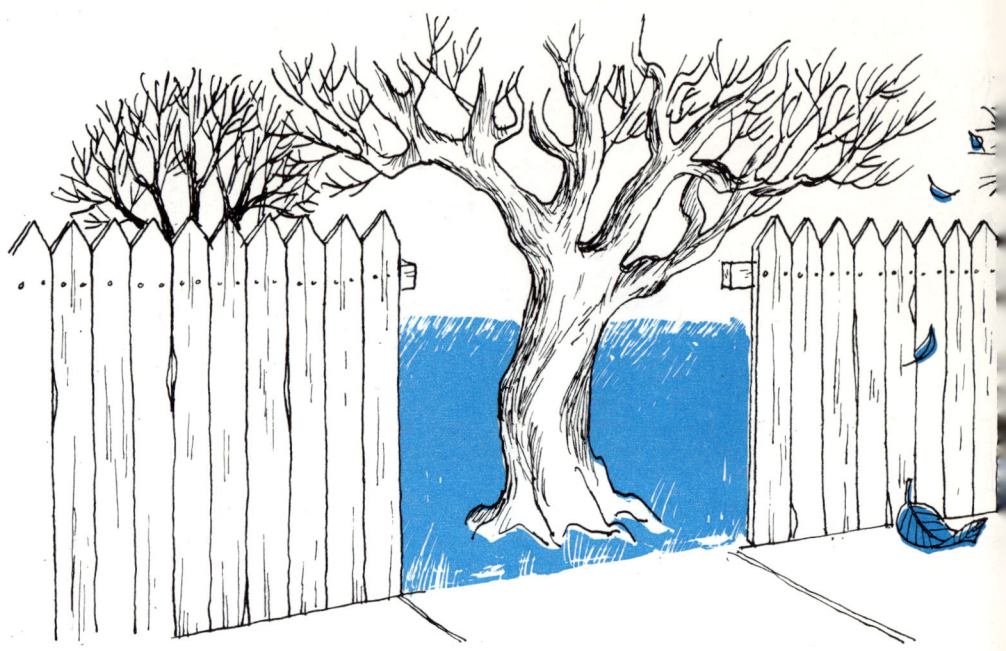

he charges for. Dad was so mad at him once that he walked out of the grocery store without paying for the meat he had in his hand. I'm not so sure he was right, either.

"But why is something right or wrong? Just saying it is doesn't make it so."

———————

Don was usually perched on the edge of his seat during the arithmetic lesson. This was one part of the school day he really liked. English had too many rules, history had too many places, and spelling had too many mistakes. But arithmetic was different.

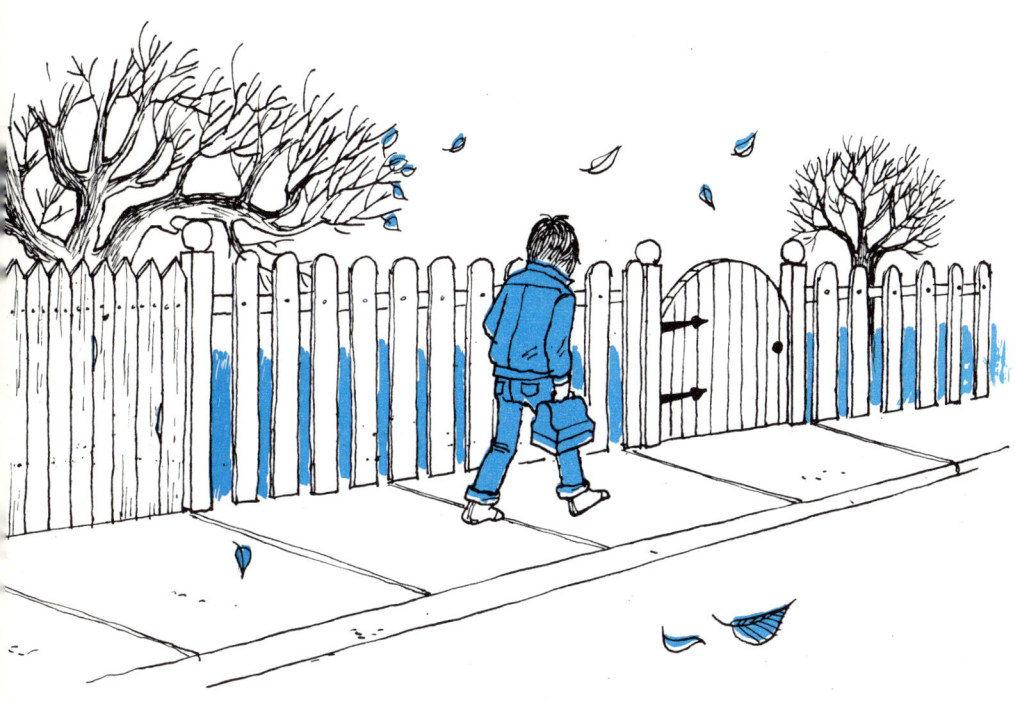

With it you could figure how long it would take to save money for a new bicycle or—some day—how long it would take to reach the moon. Arithmetic was the best period in the whole day except, of course, for recess.

Today, however, the arithmetic period was different. Don was sitting on the edge of his seat. He was watching Miss Crandall more closely than ever before; but he was not hearing a word she said. Don was thinking harder than he had ever thought. He was thinking about what Miss Crandall had said that morning before school began.

Don had come to school earlier than usual—even before his friends had finished their breakfasts. He had come early to tell Miss Crandall about the spelling test the day before. The walk to school had never seemed so short. He was at the front door and in Miss Crandall's room long before he wanted to be.

As Don sat now in arithmetic class, the whole picture of what had happened an hour earlier went through his mind:

"Don," Miss Crandall had said, "you're a human being. A human being is the most wonderful living thing we know. Think for a moment of the wonderful things you can do.

"You can talk and run and jump and play ball. How wonderful to be able to do all that!

"You can add, subtract, divide, and think things out. You can draw space ships and airplanes and even find the distance to the moon. How wonderful to do all that!

"You can bring happiness to your father and mother, have fun with your friends, and love your old brown dog, Woofer. How wonderful to do all that!

"When you are older, you can build huge buildings or be a skillful doctor or a good baseball player. A human being can do a hundred, million, trillion wonderful things!

"The people down at the church where you and I go say

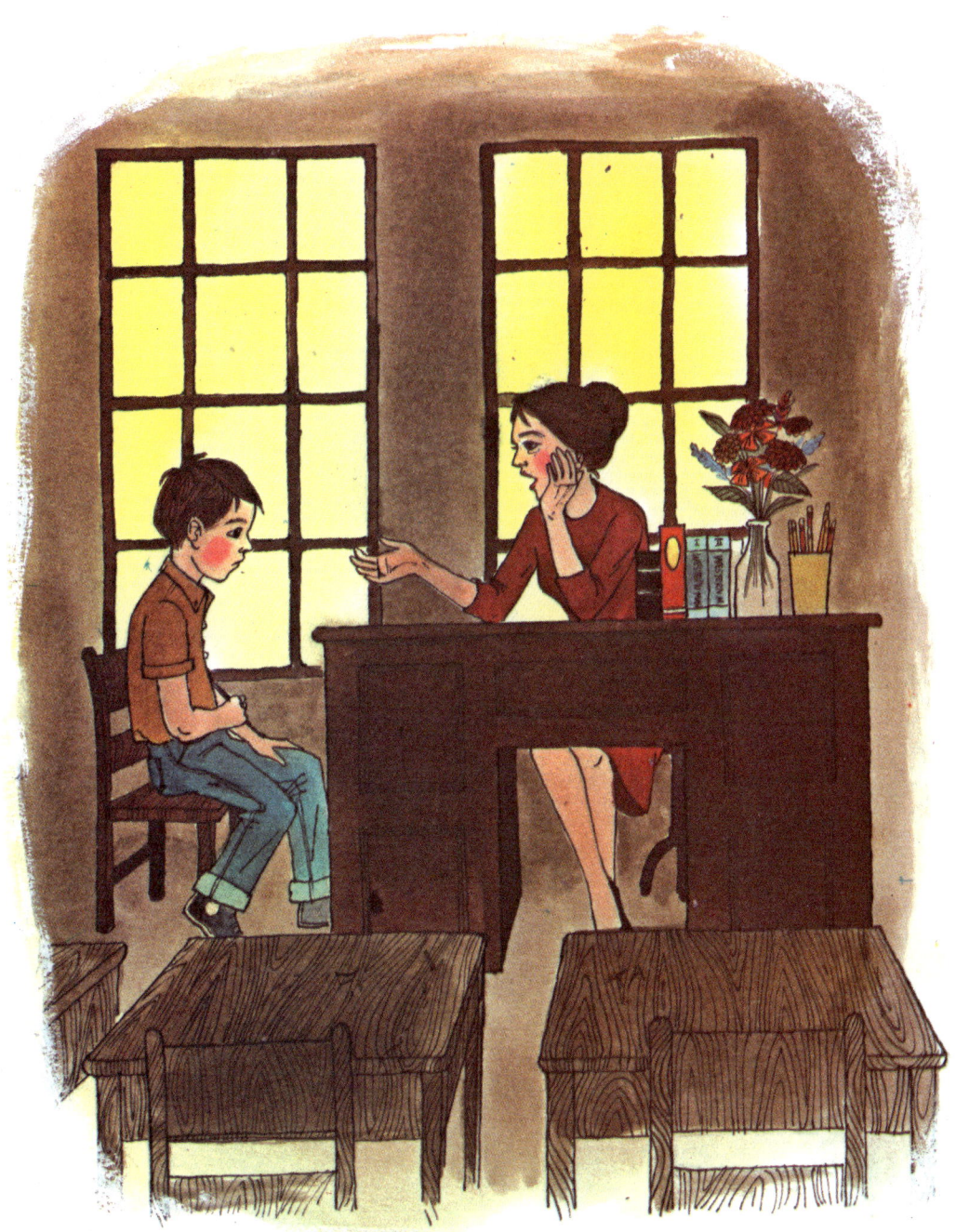

that a human being is sacred—a child of God. That's another way of saying that a human being is a most wonderful kind of living thing.

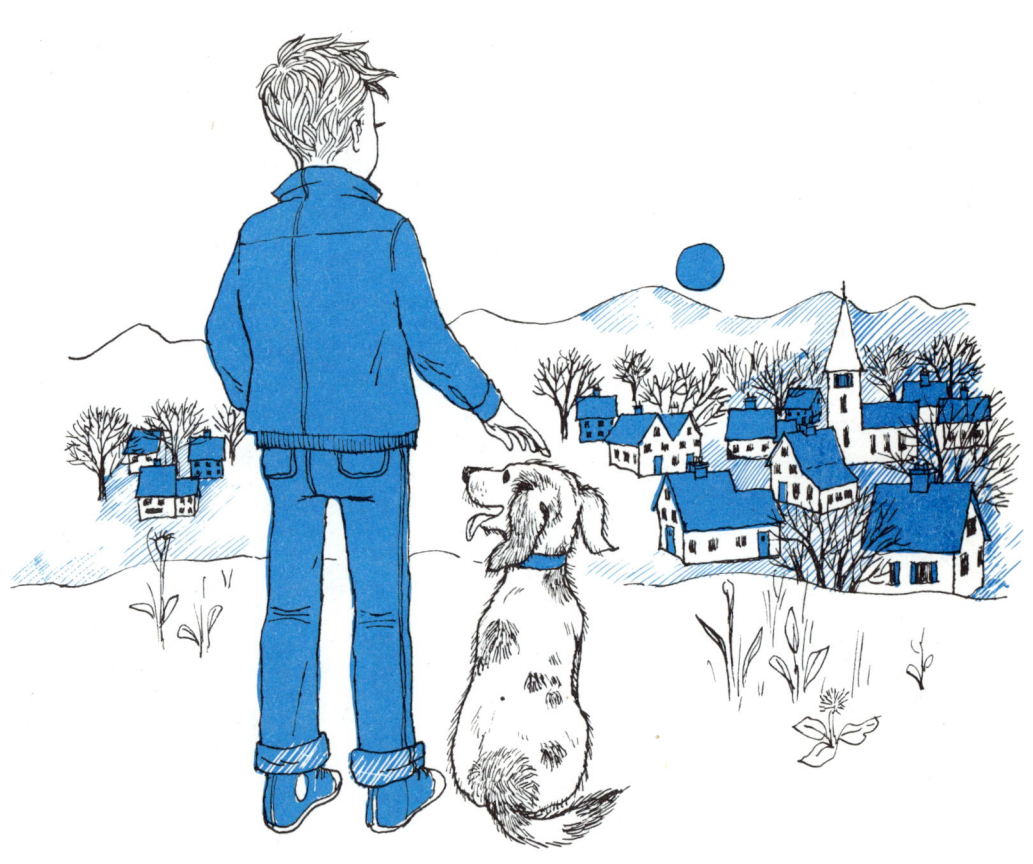

"Because a human being is such a wonderful kind of living thing, we say that something is right if it helps a human being to do the wonderful things he can do. We say that something is wrong if it stops a human being from doing the wonderful things he can do.

"One of the reasons copying on a spelling test is wrong is because a human being is not learning to do one of the most wonderful things he can do. He is not learning to speak, read, or write a language. He is not learning the words that are necessary to think and talk and write."

As Don sat there in the arithmetic class, he had an idea. "Yes," he said to himself, "a human being is the most wonderful living thing we know. To help a human being to do the wonderful things he can do is good. To stop him is wrong."

Then Don added in his thoughts, "When you talk with Miss Crandall, you feel you are one of these wonderful human beings. When you talk with Miss Crandall, you really want to do the wonderful things a human being can do. Next time," Don promised himself, "I will know that spelling lesson."

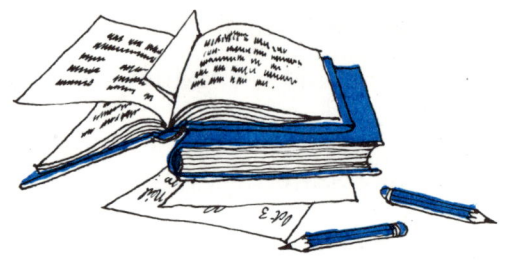

    Because spelling was not easy for Don he thought it was perhaps all right to cheat. He didn't want to get a low grade.

    Miss Crandall helped him to see that he was the person who would be hurt most if he did this. Don decided he wanted to use his own mind to do the wonderful things it was meant to do.

    I think God wants you to use your mind to do all the wonderful things a person can do.

    I think that deep down inside yourself you want to learn to do all the wonderful things you can do.

    I hope you will use your mind to do the best work you can.

                                          Larry

THE Outsider

Dear Pam and Sam:

    I think God wants you to become a person who trusts himself.

    I think that deep down inside yourself you want to become a person who trusts himself.

    What do I mean?

    Let me tell you about Sharon and the hard time she had trusting herself.

"I just don't know what to do. I simply don't know what to do! I simply do not know *what* to do!" The words came again and again from Sharon's lips. Each time she sounded a bit more desperate.

If there was one thing Sharon wanted more than anything else, it was to be one of the gang of girls in her class at school. That is, she wanted that more than anything else except one thing. Even more than she wanted to be one of the gang, Sharon wanted to be herself. She wanted to do the things she felt, deep down inside herself, she must do.

Sharon had strange feelings inside herself—at least the other girls in the gang thought they were strange. Sharon liked to be

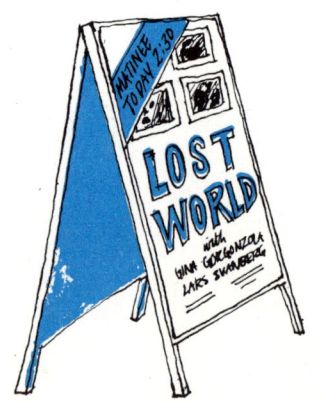
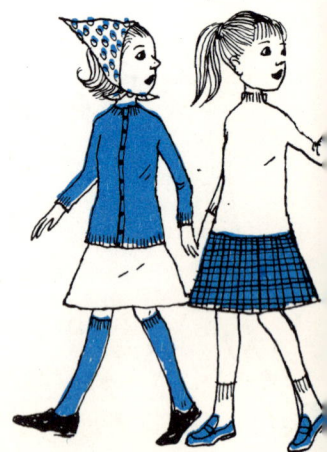

alone sometimes. She liked to go up to her room, away from everybody else, to think her thoughts and to draw.

Yes, to draw. Sharon liked to draw better than anything else she did. Especially on Friday night, after being in school all week, being with the girls, her teacher, her parents, Sharon liked to get away from everybody and go to her room and draw. Some of Sharon's drawings were pretty good! Miss Murphy, her teacher, said they were good. "Some day," Sharon thought to herself, "some day maybe I will draw even better, draw something really good."

But right now Sharon felt terrible. "I just don't know what to do," she said again. Sharon thought about the gang—Margie

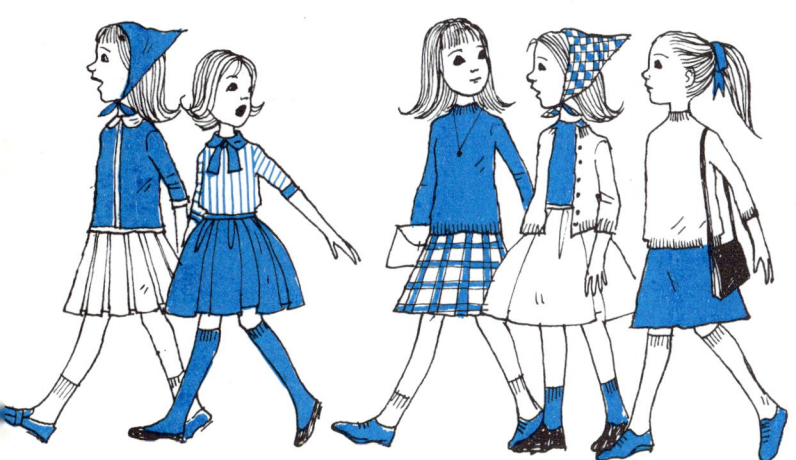

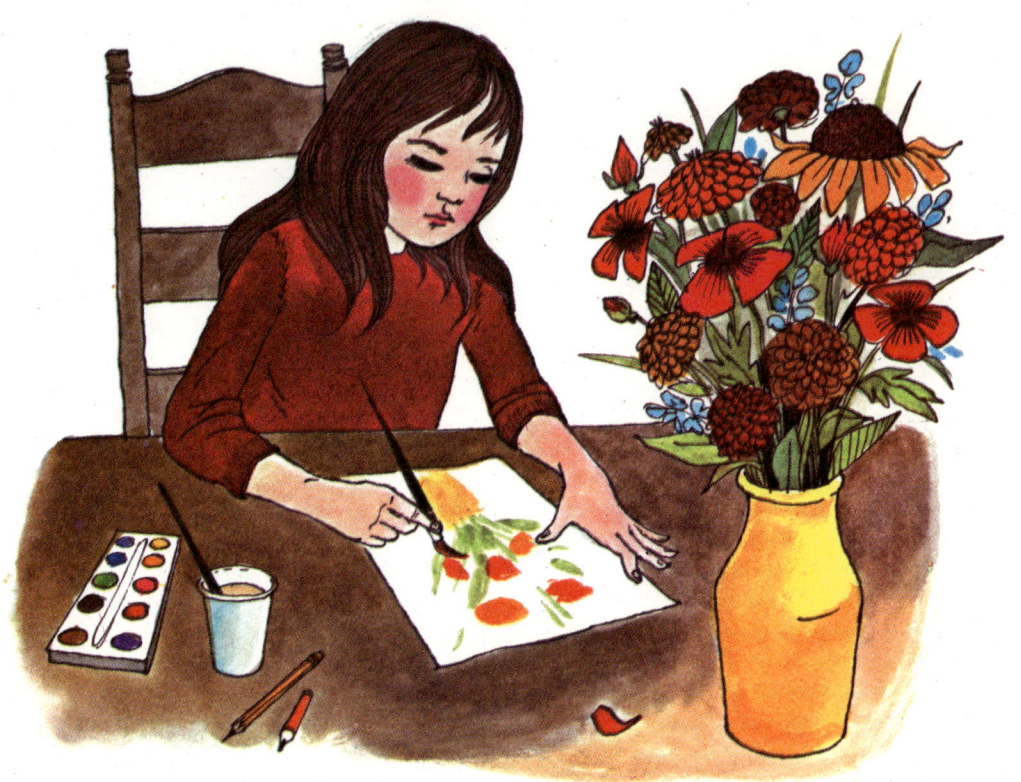

and Joan and Barbara and Jane. They were the best friends Sharon had ever known. They were really fun. There was always something going on with that gang.

Whenever you saw one, you saw all of them. They sat together at lunch time. They got together at the drugstore for cokes after school. They went to the movies together, had bunk parties at each other's houses. They were always doing something that was exciting and fun.

Next to drawing, Sharon would rather belong to this gang

than anything else. And she could be one of the gang too.

The girls wanted her, they really did. But they wanted Sharon to be with them all the time, just as they were with each other all the time.

They wanted Sharon to walk home with them after school. They wanted her to do something with them every Friday night. On Saturday mornings they played together in one of their homes, and went to the movies together Saturday afternoons. They wanted Sharon to do this too. They even went to church school together in the same car on Sunday morning. If Sharon wanted to be one of them, she would have to do all these things. She would always have to be with the gang doing things together.

It did not work unless she was with them every minute. Yesterday, for instance, Sharon called up Margie to see if she and the rest of the girls were going to the movie. They were, and Margie had said Sharon could go along. But Sharon did not really have any fun. The rest of the girls were so close that Sharon felt left out. They talked about the fun they had had at Jane's house Friday night and the bike ride they had taken that afternoon.

Finally Joan asked Sharon what she had done the night before. "I went up to my room and drew pictures," Sharon answered in a low voice.

"All by yourself?" asked Jane.

"Sure," Sharon said, "I always go off by myself to draw."

The girls were very quiet. They had strange looks on their faces.

Now it was Sunday morning. "I just don't know what to do! I just don't know," Sharon said aloud. "I want to belong to that group of girls. I want to do the things that will make them like me. But I want to be myself too. I want to think and draw all by myself. I just have to draw."

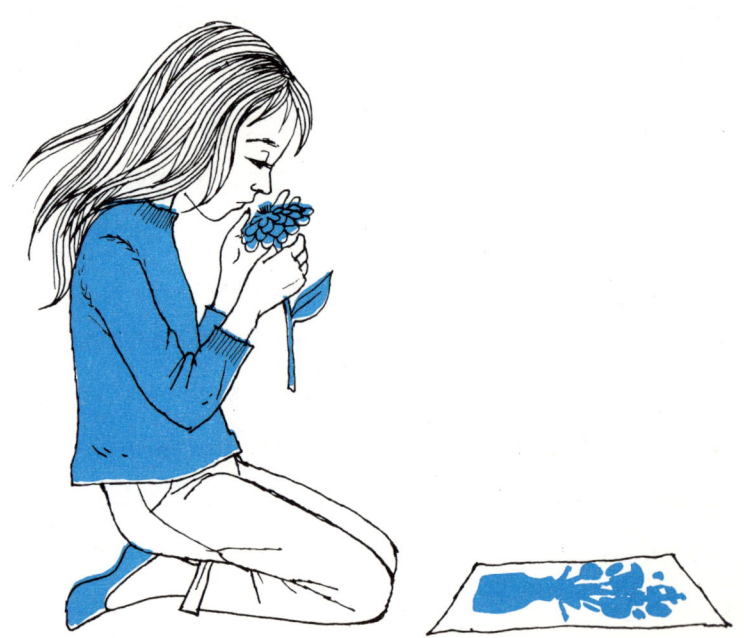

Sharon has a hard time trusting herself.

Deep down inside Sharon has an urge to draw. She wants to have fun with the gang too, but part of the time she wants to draw. Her friends do not seem to want to be alone, to draw, or do anything separately. They would rather be together almost every hour of the day.

The other girls do not understand Sharon. Because they do not understand Sharon, she thinks perhaps there is something strange about herself. She thinks there is something strange about wanting to draw. She does not trust herself. She does not trust her own feelings.

I think God wants you to become a person who trusts himself. I think God wants you to learn to trust the thoughts and feelings inside you.

I think you want to trust yourself. I think you want to be a person who trusts the feelings and thoughts inside yourself.

I hope you become a person who trusts himself.

Larry

Susy looks for ANSWERS

Dear Pam and Sam:

I think God wants you to become a thoughtful person.

I think that deep down inside yourself you want to become a thoughtful person.

What do I mean?

In my first letter to you I wrote about God who is able to make a human being. One of the wonderful things about a human being is that he can think. He can think about the things that happen to him. He can try to understand these things. He can try to understand the world in which he lives.

Not long ago I knew a girl named Susy. Like many third- and fourth-grade boys and girls she wondered about prayer. Before she could understand even a little bit, however, she had to do some thinking. She had to do some hard thinking.

Let me tell you a story about what Susy learned about prayer. The story has several parts.

Susy eyed the beautiful blue taffeta dress in Carlson's shop window. "Oh, boy," she murmured under her breath, "just what I want for Beverly's party Friday night. Wait until I tell Mom."

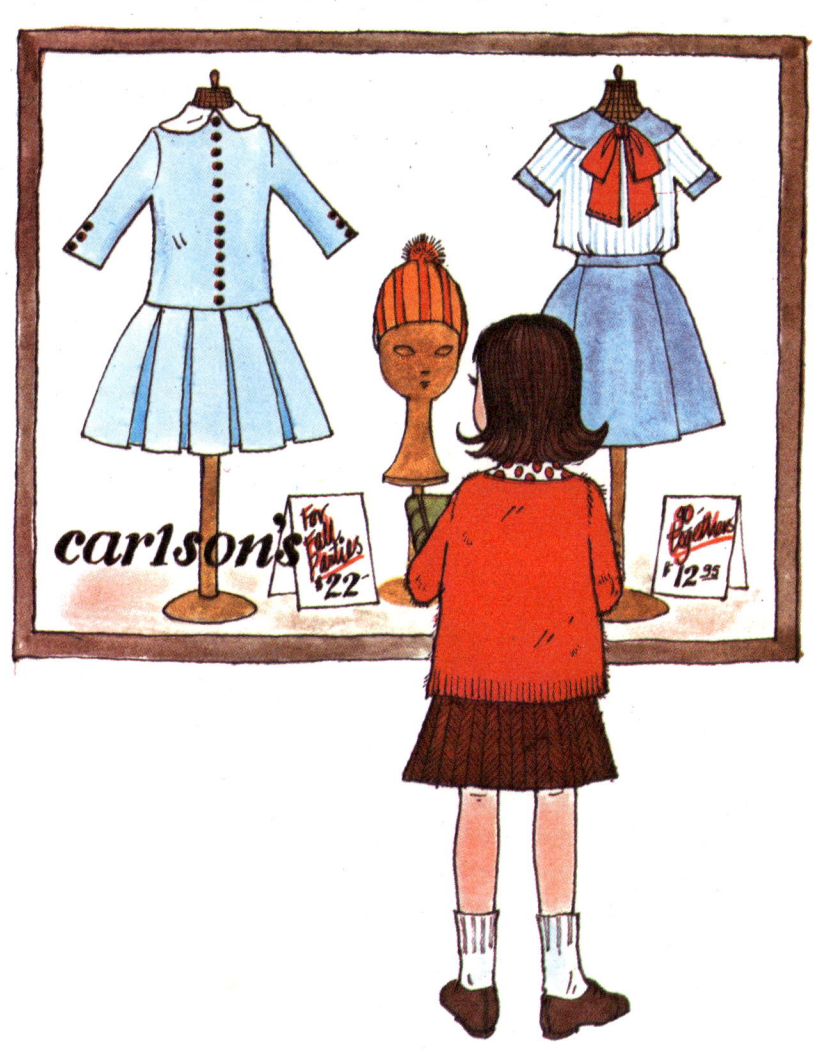

Susy cut across three back yards in order to get home quicker. "Hey, Mom," she shouted as she flung open the kitchen door. "Hey, Mom, did you see the dress at Carlson's? It's blue with lots of red buttons and a white Peter Pan collar. It's really neat and I'd like to have it for Beverly's party. Can I, Mom, can I?"

"Wait a minute," said Susy's mother, "what just hit the house, a cyclone?"

"No, no, it's me," said Susy. "Can I, Mom, can I?"

"Well, Susy, I don't know," answered her mother. "You know we have a clothes budget and I don't think we planned on a new dress this month for you, at least not one that costs as much as the one you described. You had better ask your dad."

"Dad, Dad," shouted Susy as he drove into the driveway. Hopping into the car even before Dad had a chance to get out, Susy tried to say ten words at the same time.

"Hold on," said her dad. "Who wound you up and put a nickel in? Now what's on your mind?"

"Dad, I want the new dress in Carlson's," replied Susy. "You should see it. It's real neat and blue and has a Peter Pan collar. I could wear it to Beverly's party and I wouldn't ask for another dress ever, and I . . ."

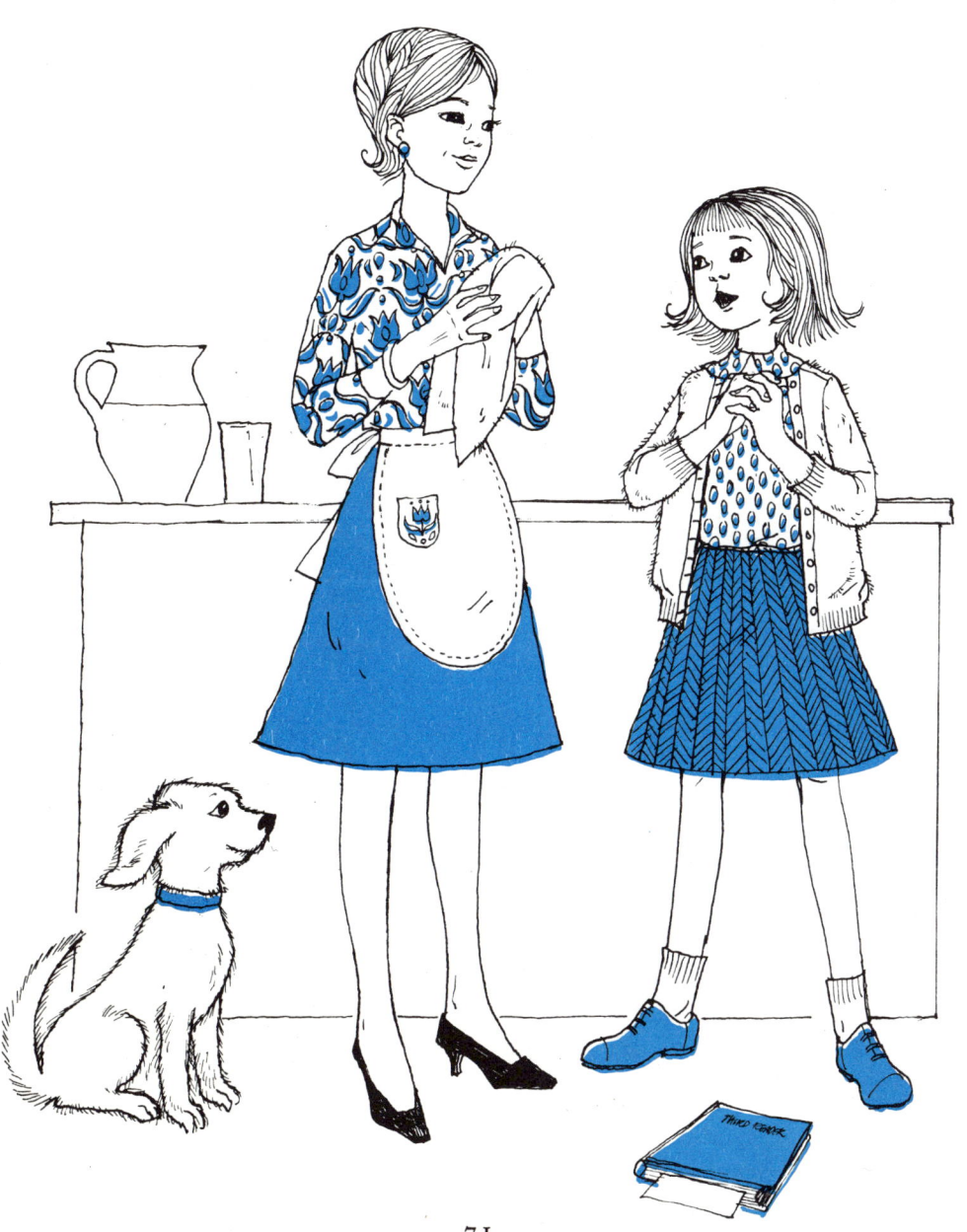

Ten minutes later Susy and Dad got out of the car. Susy guessed Dad was right. She had had her share of the clothes budget for the time being. She did have another party dress she had worn only twice but she did want that dress she saw in Carlson's window. She really wanted it. Suddenly she had an idea.

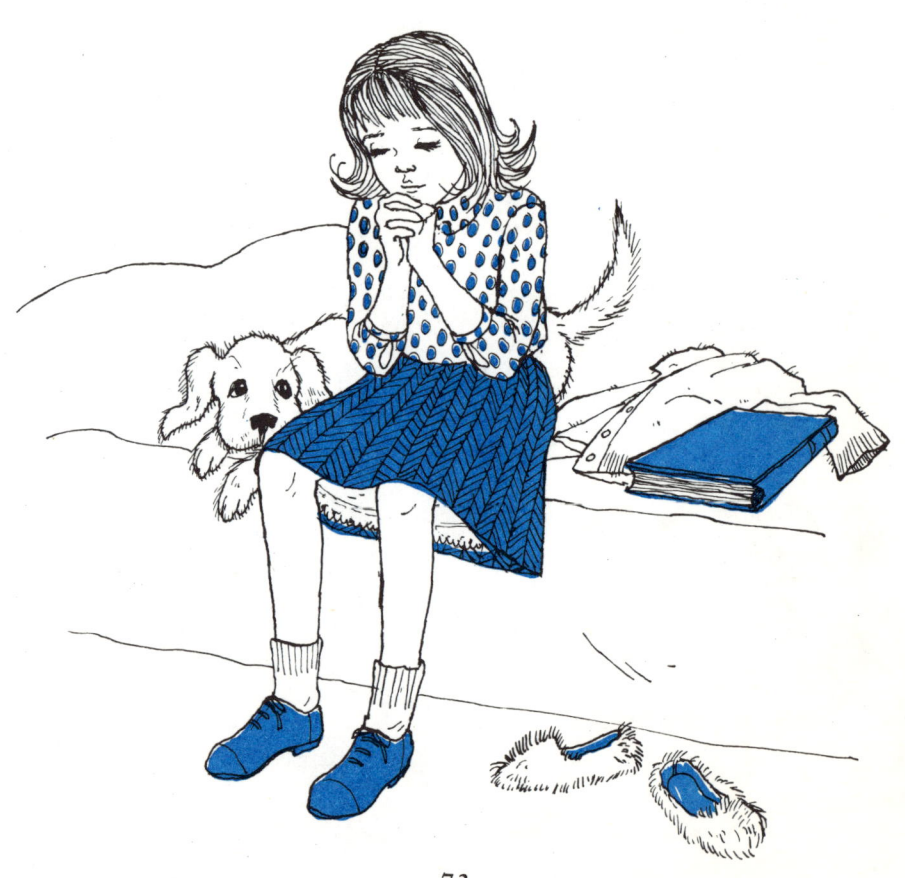

She dashed upstairs quickly, closed the door to her room, sat down on her bed and said, "Dear God, I know you can do anything. I know you hear everybody's prayers. Miss Dillon at church school said you do. Please, God, I don't know how you will do it, but please give me the dress. Please, God, please! Amen."

Susy could hardly wait until she got to church school, and that was unusual for Susy. She popped into the room like a jack-in-the-box and spied her teacher talking with Jack and Wally. Susy ran up to Miss Dillon. Susy was almost as out of breath as her dog, Boomba, after he had chased a rabbit.

"Miss Dillon," she said breathlessly. Before Miss Dillon even had a chance to say "Hello," Susy continued: "Miss Dillon, didn't you say a few weeks ago that if we really wanted something we could pray to God and he would help us get it?"

"Yes," said Miss Dillon, trying to remember what she had said and also wondering what question Susy was going to ask that would be hard to answer.

"Well," replied Susy, "I wanted a new dress this week—the one in Carlson's dress shop. I wanted it so badly I prayed and prayed, but God didn't do a thing about it. The dress is still in Carlson's window, and I had to go to Beverly's party in a dress I had already worn twice."

"Whillikers!" said Jack, before Miss Dillon could reply. "Just like a girl to have such a silly idea. I prayed for a baseball mitt when I was a little kid but my mom says you can't expect a baseball mitt to jump out of a store window just because you ask God to give it to you. Prayer doesn't do things like that. What a silly idea!"

"I didn't ask you," said Susy, giving Jack a look that would have withered a dandelion. "What do you think, Miss Dillon?"

Miss Dillon said, "Susy, let's take time enough today in our class to think this through. You tell the whole class what you have just told me and we will see what ideas each of us has."

An hour later Susy trudged toward home. What a lot of thoughts she had twirling around in her head! Susy puzzled slowly over each one of them. She remembered what Jack had said about praying for things.

Marilyn had a different idea. She thought you could pray for things, but only if they were for someone else. Susy wondered about this. If she had asked God to give the dress to Mary Foster who did not have many dresses, would God have given it to Mary?

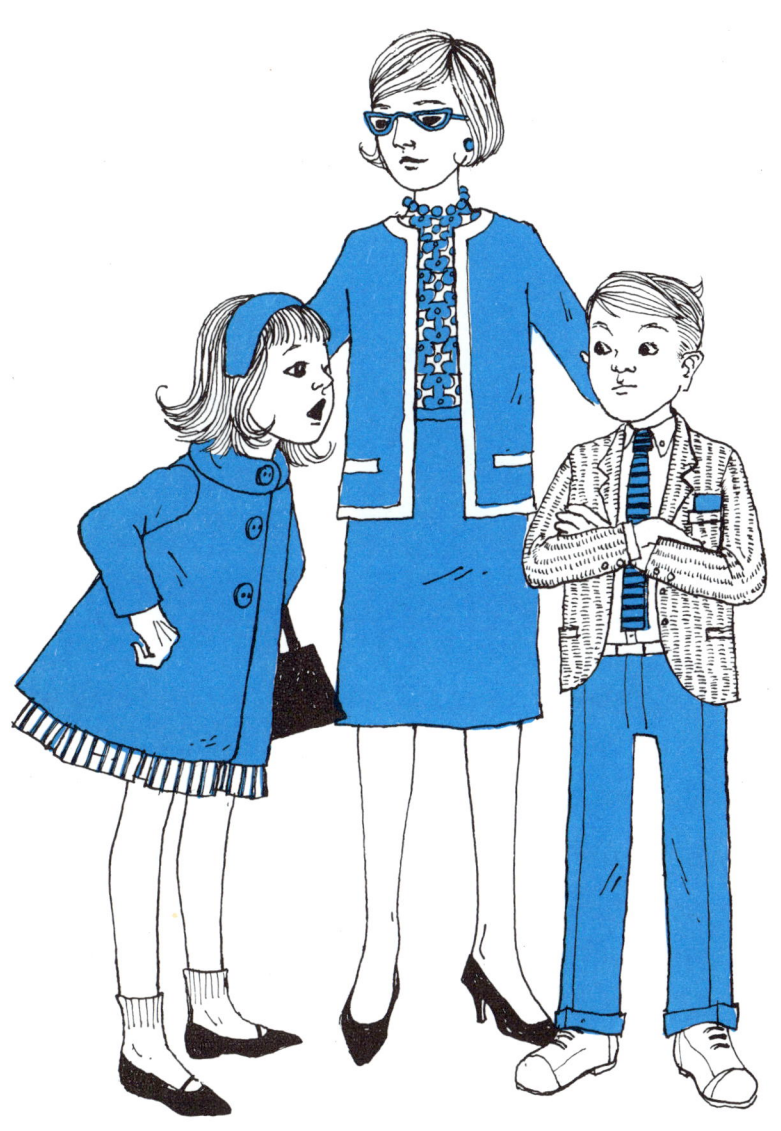

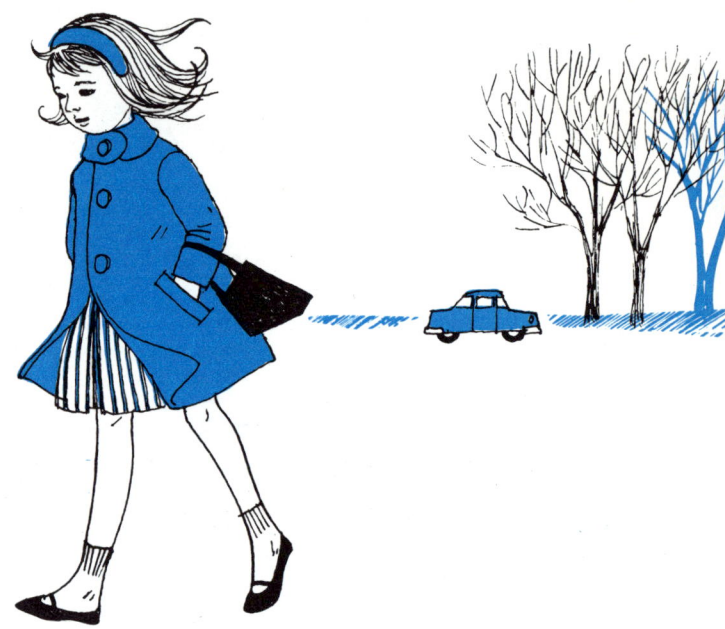

Miss Dillon said that when she thought of praying for *things* she tried to remember the Lord's prayer. Jesus taught us to pray "Give us this day our daily bread." It is right to ask God to help us whenever we need help.

Finally Susy thought about Wally's remark. He said God gives people minds with which to think and bodies with which to work. Wally did not think God reached down and handed out dresses when someone prayed for them.

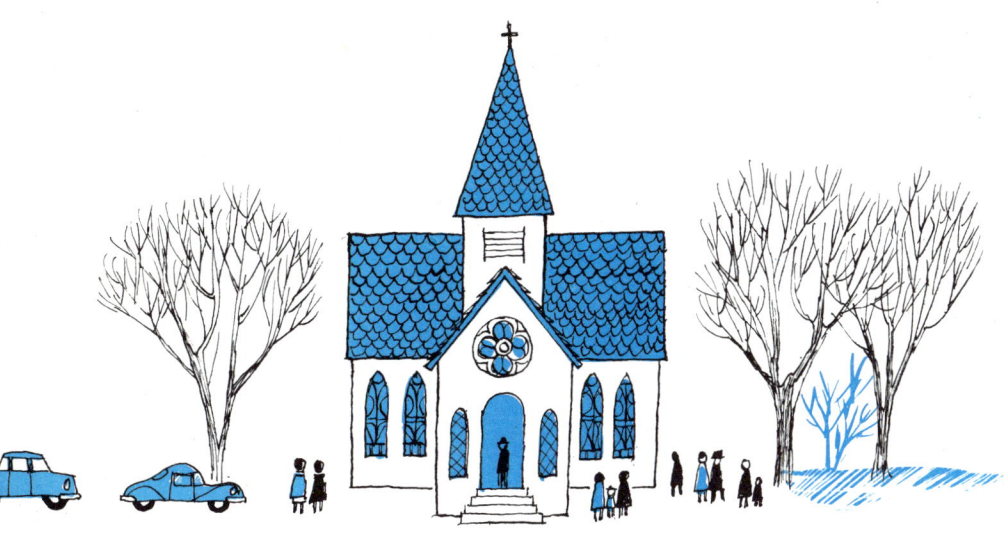

    Miss Dillon seemed to understand how much Susy had wanted the dress. She said, "It isn't always possible for God to give us exactly what we ask for. But he understands how much you wanted the blue dress. You may find he is giving another kind of answer to your prayer. His love will help you to meet the disappointment. He wants us to trust him to give us the best possible answer to our prayers."

    Susy felt better as she thought over all that had been said. But she still did not understand everything about prayer.

So many exciting things had happened at school during the week that Susy had almost forgotten her questions about prayer and the dress in Carlson's store. On the way home from school the day before she had looked in the window of the store and noticed that the dress was gone. But Beverly's party was almost a week ago and Susy never worried about things that had happened in the past. She was quite happy as she skipped home from school Friday afternoon with the whole weekend before her. She was going to Lynn's for a birthday supper that night and to the movies on Saturday afternoon.

But when Susy reached home, her dad was at the door with the news that her mother was very, very sick. He had taken her to the hospital a few hours before. Mother would probably be well in a few weeks, but she would have an operation first thing in the morning and would be in the hospital for several days.

Dinner that evening at Susy's house was a quiet affair. Susy wasn't hungry nor were her father and her older sister Tina. Seating themselves at the table the family bowed their heads for a moment of silence. Susy, her dad and mom and Tina always did this before eating together. It was a time to thank God for food and for the many people who spend their lives growing it and preparing it for eating.

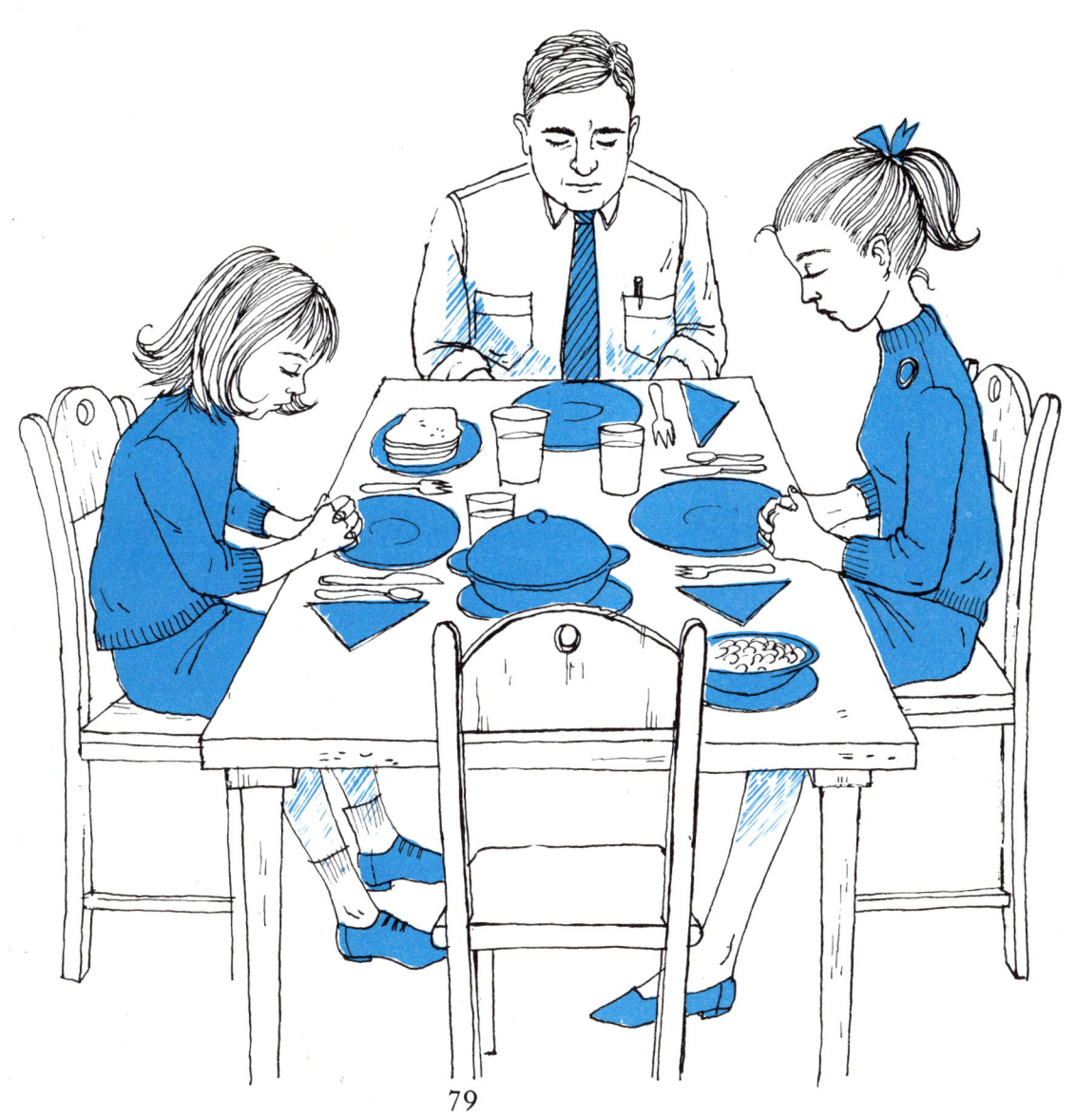

That evening, however, they had other thoughts on their minds. Susy's father knew what they were all thinking. He said, "Dear God, please be very near to Mother in the hospital. Be near to each of us while Mother is away. Help us to be strong and brave while we are without her. Amen."

Susy looked up through tearful eyes toward her father. Then she almost shouted, "And dear God, please don't let Mommy have to have the operation. Please let her come home tomorrow."

Her father looked at her and said, "We miss Mother very much, don't we?"

Later that evening Susy's father was troubled. He could understand Susy's prayer tonight. But last week Susy believed that God would answer her prayer for a dress. Tonight it almost seemed as if Susy thought God would reach down the next day and send her mother home well and happy without an operation.

He wondered about Susy's prayer. He wondered what she thought about prayer. Of one thing her father was certain. He wanted to talk with Susy soon about prayer.

Two weeks later Susy was stretched out on the old rug in front of the fireplace. Her dad was getting settled in his favorite chair. The evening would have been perfect if her mother had been there, but at least Susy had her father all to herself. Her

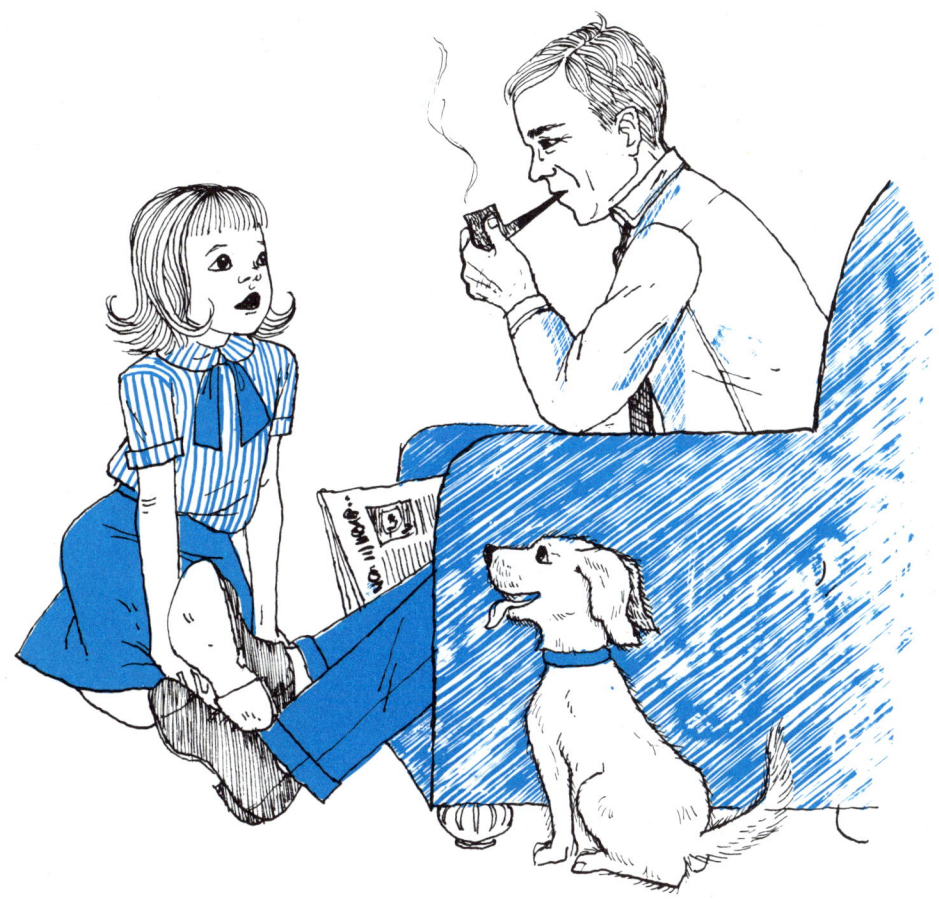

sister had left to spend the evening with her friend Janet. Most of the time Susy thought her sister was absolutely the best, but every now and then it was really wonderful to have her father all to herself.

Susy was about to suggest a game of Monopoly when her father suddenly asked, "Susy, what do you think God is like?"

Sitting up from her stretched-out position and tucking her feet under her, Susy gave him a long, puzzled look. "I don't know," she said. "I really don't know. I used to think he was a friend—someone who helped you get things you wanted or saw that things worked out the way you wanted them to. I'll never think that again, though."

"You mean because of the dress and because of what happened to Mother?" asked Susy's dad.

"Yes," said Susy. "I asked God for the dress and didn't get it. I could understand about that when Miss Dillon said we shouldn't pray for things we don't really need. Then I asked God to make Mother well so she would not have to have the operation. Instead, she had to have part of one of her lungs taken out. Yesterday you said we would never be able to go to our cabin in the mountains again because breathing would be too hard for Mother in the high mountains. Mother is getting well,

I know, and will be coming home next week. Still, God certainly didn't make things turn out the way I wanted them."

Her father sounded thoughtful as he said, "I don't understand everything about prayer either, Susy. Perhaps the best part about all of this is that you are asking questions and thinking about them. I believe God loves us, and that he wants us to have what is best for us. We must learn to love him enough to trust his answers. Sometimes these cannot be exactly what we ask for.

"You and I are ever so grateful that Mother is well enough to be coming home, even if she can't do everything she could do before. Through all of this experience we have felt God's nearness and his love, giving us strength to meet whatever comes."

Susy's face was still puzzled. "Are there some things God can't do, then?" she asked.

Her father hesitated before he answered, for this was an even harder question.

"Susy," he said, "God has created a dependable world with laws in it that determine how things can happen and how they can't. From all I have been able to see and observe, God works through these laws."

"But God could create a dress if he really wanted to, couldn't he?" asked Susy.

"Before a dress can be created, the cotton, or other material, must be grown according to God's laws for plant life. Cotton is then made into cloth and into dresses on machines that run according to the laws of physics. The growing of the cotton, the making of the cloth into dresses, seem to require the help of man. I really doubt if God would by-pass all this and create a dress to give to a girl named Susy."

"I suppose that is right," said Susy, "but let me ask you one more thing. Couldn't God put an idea in your mind to buy me the dress?"

Her dad threw a great big grin at Susy. "You know," he said, "I think God is very near us urging us to care for other people and to help each other. But I doubt if God is urging every father and mother to go out and buy every dress or baseball mitt that their children want."

"But I thought . . ." Susy started to reply when the telephone rang. She ran to the hallway to answer it. In half a minute she returned shouting to her dad, "It's Mom! She's a little lonesome at the hospital and wants to talk with us. Come on!" With a sigh of relief Susy's dad hurried toward the telephone.

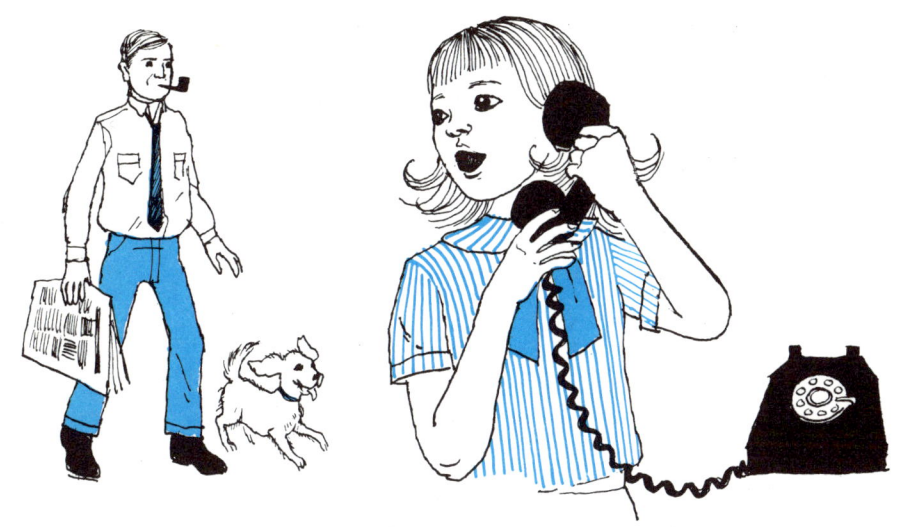

Susy did not usually think to bring in the morning paper. This morning the paper boy's throw was wild and the paper banged hard on the big picture window in the living room. Susy could not help noticing that the paper had arrived.

She almost changed her mind about bringing it in when she opened the door. The cold air came rushing in upon her, but she held her breath and made a quick dash across the porch and picked up the paper. Spreading it out on the table, she was about to turn to the funnies when something on the front page caught her eye. The headline said: "Dog Lost, Small Girl Prays for Eight Months, Dog Found."

Up the stairs dashed Susy, faster than she ever went when her parents called her. Almost slipping on the small rug in the upstairs hall, she fairly zoomed into her father's bedroom. He had just finished struggling with the collar button on his shirt and was making the first loop in tying his tie.

"Look, Dad," shouted Susy with what little breath she had left. "It does work! Prayer does work! Right here on the front page—a girl lost her dog eight months ago and prayed every night that it would come back. Yesterday someone found it and the little girl has it back. What do you think of that? Prayer does work!"

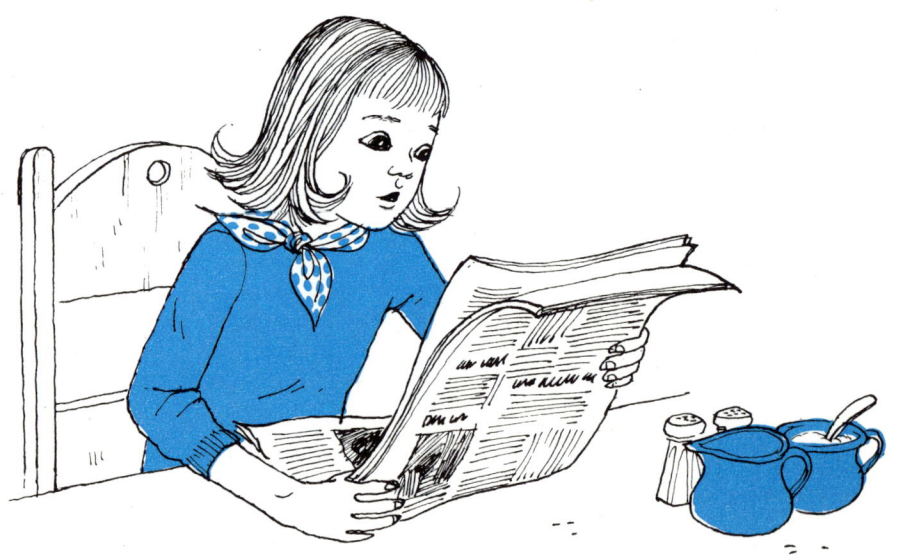

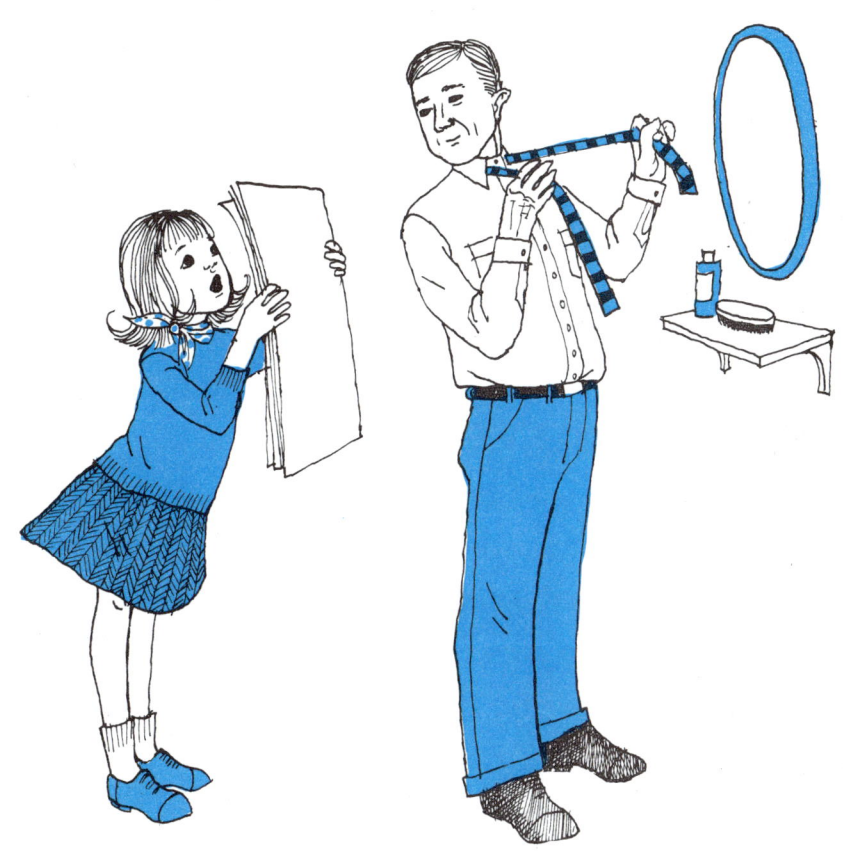

Susy's dad took a hurried look at his watch but then a thought came to him. "O.K.," he thought, "I'll be late to work this morning." He sat down on the side of the bed. "Susy," he said, "I'm not trying to convince you one way or the other on your questions about prayer. I only want you to hear different opinions and different people's experiences. Then be as careful as you can in making up your own mind."

"But it says it right here," replied Susy. "A girl lost her dog. She prayed for it every night for eight months. Now it has come back. Doesn't that prove that prayer works?"

"How about the thousands of boys and girls who have lost their dogs and prayed that they would come back but they never did?" asked her father.

"Well, I don't know," said Susy, "but some of my friends say that when you pray for God to do something and he doesn't do it, it's because God is doing what he thinks is best for you."

"That's an interesting idea, Susy," said her father. "If you think God decides these things anyway, why pray?"

"Hmm, I don't know," puzzled Susy, whose head was in a whirl. "Why do you think the little girl's dog came back?"

"To be perfectly honest with you, Susy, I don't really believe that what was best for her, or prayer, had anything to do with it. I think life is like that. Dogs wander away and get lost. Sometimes they are found and brought back. Sometimes they are found and kept. Sometimes they get hurt and die. Sometimes they wander around for years. That is the way life is. God has been able to create this wonderful form of life we call a dog but he does not decide everything that happens to each one."

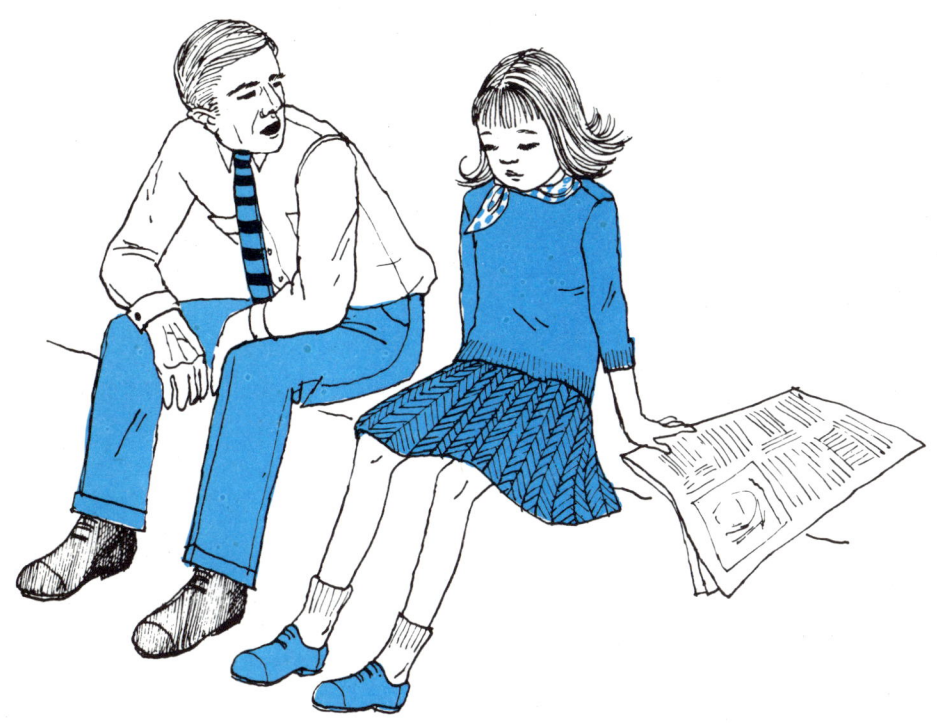

By now Susy was thinking back over other questions she still had about prayer. "You know," she said, "we never did talk about whether my asking God for Mother to come home the next day could make any difference. I suppose you don't think that helps either."

Looking toward the window her father slowly searched his thoughts. "I believe," he said, "that if Mother had known you were praying for her it might have helped. I believe that if we had gone to the hospital and prayed with her it might have helped. I think if we prayed that her doctor and surgeon would know how to do what her body needed it might have helped.

"You see, I think that God is always very near to us, wanting to help us if we will let him. I think that God is always very near wanting to share his strength and courage with us. I think praying with Mother might have helped her to find the strength and courage which God wants to share with her.

"God can help us be strong and courageous when we are sick. He can help us keep trying to get well. But this does not happen just by someone closing her eyes and saying, 'Please, God, don't let Mommy have to have an operation.' It happens, when it does, when we really struggle to find the courage and strength of God and when we really struggle to overcome our illness.

"I do believe that God expects us to ask him to help those whom we love, and others whom we do not know, too. He wants us to pray for each other.

"When we ask for things we cannot have, I believe God gives us courage and strength to meet the disappointment. He helps us to feel his love close around us.

"We can love and trust God, for he is our Father. We can be sure he will answer our prayers in the best way possible.

"And now, Susy, if I don't get to work I'm going to be in more trouble than a dog lost for eight months. I'll see you this afternoon. Hurry home from school because we're going to get Mother at the hospital and bring her home."

"Don't worry about me," shouted Susy with a joy that answered every question for the moment. "I'll be here. Just don't be late."

Susy's dad grinned as he drove off. He had quite a daughter and he hoped she would keep searching all her life the way she was searching now.

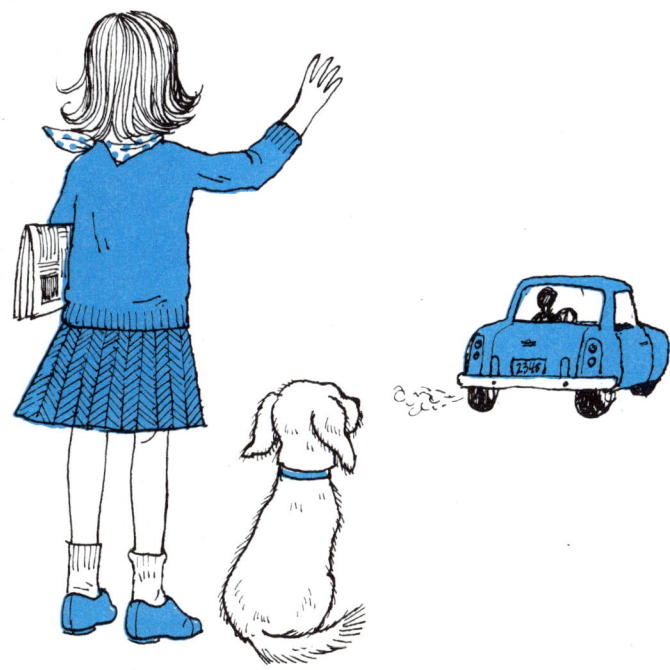

Susy was becoming a thoughtful person. She was thinking about the things that happened to her and to other people. She was trying to understand these things. Her mind was filled with questions for which she was seeking answers.

It may take Susy a long time to find answers that satisfy her. She may not ever find the answers to some questions. But a thoughtful person keeps on searching.

I think God wants you to become a thoughtful person. I think God wants you to keep thinking and searching for right answers.

I think that deep down inside yourself you want to be a thoughtful person. I think you really want to keep searching to find answers that seem right to you.

I hope you become a thoughtful person.

Larry

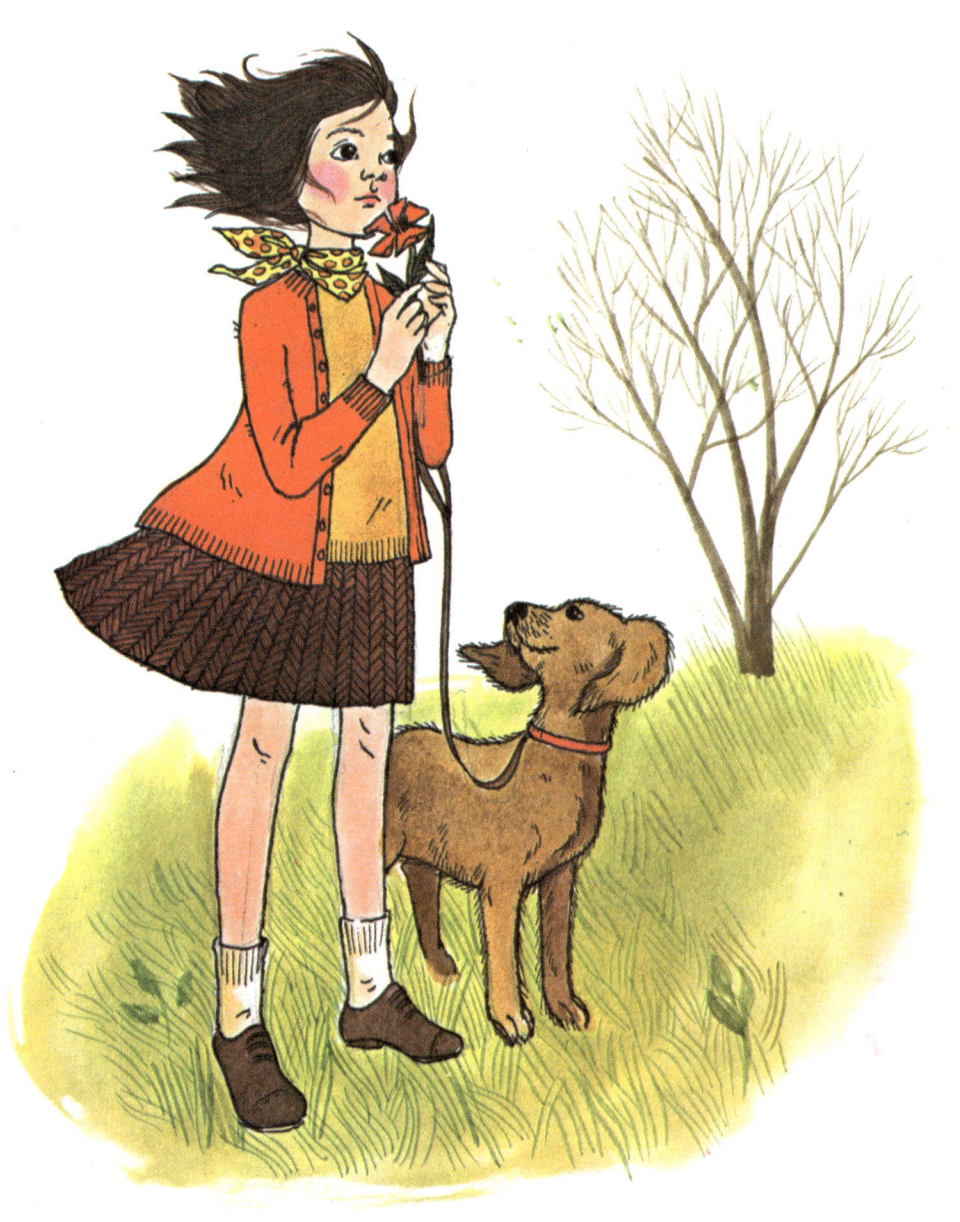

Dear Pam and Sam:

I would like to end this book with a prayer. Read it slowly again and again. I hope that all through the year you will find this a helpful prayer. Think about it as you read it.

Dear God, help me to trust myself. Help me to trust the feelings and thoughts inside myself after I have examined them closely.

Help me to be a person of justice. Help me to feel and think how another person feels if he is treated a certain way.

Help me to become a creative person. Help me to create something out of my own feelings and thoughts that will make the world a better place.

With God's Help

Help me to be a person of power. Help me to decide for myself what to do in a hard situation—and to do it.

Help me to be a thoughtful person. Help me to understand deeply and clearly the many things going on around me.

Help me to be able to trust others. Help me to be able to accept their love and friendship if they offer it to me.

Dear God, help me to become what I am able to become, with your help. Amen.

I hope that with God's help you become the kind of person God and you want you to become.

Larry

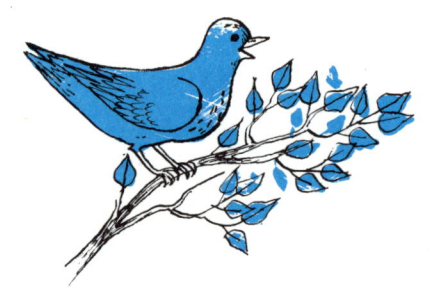